Somatic Exercises for Beginners and Weight Loss

Dive into a transformative journey with this comprehensive guide, blending somatic exercises, mindful practices, and nutritional insights to harmonize your physical and emotional well-being. Unlock the secrets to lasting health, flexibility, and inner peace through accessible, step-by-step strategies tailored for lifelong wellness.

By

Jade Quinn

COPYRIGHT © 2024 BY AUTHOR

All rights reserved.

It is illegal to reproduce, duplicate, or share any section of this document, whether in electronic or printed form. Digital recording and storage of this publication is strictly prohibited and is not permitted without the written permission of the publisher. Only the use of quotations in reviews or articles is permitted.

Table of Contents

Somatic Exercises for Beginners and Weight Loss 1

Introduction to Somatic Exercises 1
    Definition and Origins 1
    Benefits of Somatic Exercises 2
    Somatic Exercises and Weight Loss 4
    Overview of the Book 6

Chapter 1: Understanding Your Body 11
    1.1 Body Awareness: 11
    1.2 The Science of Stress and Weight: 13
    1.3 Emotional Eating and How to Address It: 14

Chapter 2: Foundations of Somatic Exercises 17
    2.1 Principles of Somatic Movement: 17
    2.2 Breathing Techniques: 18
    2.3 Posture and Alignment: 20

Chapter 3: Somatic Exercises Explained 23
    3.1 Warm-Up Movements 25
    3.2 Core Somatic Movements 50

Chapter 4: Mindful Practices for Emotional Balance 71
    4.1 Mindfulness and Meditation: 71
    4.2 Mindfulness and Meditation: 72
    4.3 Journaling for Emotional Awareness: 74
    Download your Tracking Journal for your exercises. 75

Chapter 5: Nutritional Insights for Weight Loss 77
    5.1 Basic Nutrition Principles: 77

5.2 Foods That Support Somatic Practice 79

5.3 Integrating Nutrition with Somatic Exercises 81

Chapter 6: A 4-Week Somatic Exercise Plan 83

6.1 Setting Realistic Goals: 83

6.2 Weekly Plans with Daily Exercises: 84

Week 1: Foundation and Mind-Body Connection 86

Week 2: Foundation and Mind-Body Connection 93

Week 3: Deepening Practice and Enhancing Endurance 102

Week 4: Integration and Advanced Practices 111

Chapter 7: Overcoming Challenges and Maintaining Progress 120

7.1 Common Obstacles and Strategies for Overcoming Them 120

7.2 Building a Support System 122

7.3 Sustaining Motivation and Results 123

Conclusion 126

Creating a Sustainable Routine 126

The Journey Ahead 128

Introduction to Somatic Exercises

Definition and Origins

Somatic exercises are a powerful and accessible way to improve your health and well-being by integrating the mind, body, and spirit. These exercises recognize that your body and mind are deeply interconnected, and they enhance this connection to promote better awareness and control over your physical state. Somatic exercises originated in the early 20th century and were influenced by practices like yoga, tai chi, and Feldenkrais. All of these practices share the belief that mindfulness and physical movement are crucial for unlocking your body's potential for health, balance, and transformation.

The term "somatic" itself comes from the Greek word "soma," meaning "the living body." It emphasizes your body's perceived internal experiences rather than its external appearance or movement. Somatic exercises, therefore, focus on the inner experience of action and the sensations that arise from it, such as tension, relaxation, and the flow of energy throughout your body. This approach is distinct from conventional exercise regimens that prioritize external form and performance, sometimes at the expense of self-awareness and internal harmony.

Historically, somatic practices were pioneered by individuals such as Moshé Feldenkrais, who developed the Feldenkrais Method, and Thomas Hanna, who coined the term "somatics" in the 1970s. These pioneers recognized that habitual movement patterns and posture, often developed in response to stress or injury, could lead to chronic pain and decreased mobility. They developed somatic exercises to reeducate your body and mind, teaching you to release these patterns and adopt healthier ones. Through gentle movements and focused attention, practitioners learn to increase their bodily awareness, identify areas of tension, and cultivate more efficient, graceful, and pain-free moving methods.

At its core, somatic exercise is not merely a physical practice but a holistic philosophy that acknowledges the intricate relationship between physical movement, emotional states, and mental well-being. It operates on the principle that changing how you move can change how you feel and think, leading to profound transformations in your overall health and quality of life.

As we delve into the benefits of somatic exercises in the following sections, you'll explore how this practice can help alleviate physical pain, reduce stress, enhance emotional balance, and foster a deeper connection with your body. These exercises offer more than just physical benefits; they are a gateway to understanding your body's responses and needs, allowing you to overcome physical and emotional barriers. You can achieve a harmonious balance between mind and body through the mindful practice of bodily exercises, unlocking the potential for lasting health, flexibility, and strength.

As you progress through this book, you will learn about the history and theoretical basis of somatic exercises and discover practical applications that can be incorporated into your daily life. This comprehensive approach aims to balance physical and emotional well-being by providing tools such as mindful practices that promote emotional balance and nutritional insights that support physical health. By doing so, you can embark on an enlightening journey of self-discovery and healing.

Benefits of Somatic Exercises

In the realm of health and fitness, weight loss is often a primary goal for many individuals. Yet, the journey to losing weight is not merely about the numbers on a scale; it encompasses a holistic approach that nurtures both the body and mind. This is where somatic exercises shine, offering a unique pathway to weight loss that transcends traditional exercise methods by fostering a deep, mindful connection with one's body. This section delves into how somatic exercises can be a powerful ally in achieving weight loss and enhancing overall well-being, seamlessly linking this concept with the comprehensive exploration of the book.

Somatic exercises, with their emphasis on mindful movement and body awareness, offer a nuanced approach to weight loss. Instead of focusing on high-intensity workouts that can often lead to burnout or injury, these practices encourage a gentle, sustainable path to physical health. By engaging in somatic exercises, individuals learn to listen to their bodies, recognizing signs of hunger, fullness, stress, and relaxation. This heightened awareness can lead to more mindful eating patterns and a reduction in stress-related eating, which are crucial factors in managing weight.

Moreover, somatic exercises contribute to weight loss by improving metabolic function and body composition. As these exercises enhance flexibility, posture, and muscle tone, they also increase efficiency in movement. This improvement in physical functioning can boost metabolism, helping the body to burn calories more effectively even when at rest. Additionally, the stress-reducing properties of somatic practices can lower levels of cortisol, a hormone that not only contributes to weight gain, particularly in the abdominal area but also affects overall health negatively.

Beyond the physical aspects, somatic exercises offer profound emotional and mental health benefits that support weight loss journeys. Stress, anxiety, and negative body image can be significant barriers to weight loss. Through the mindful practice of somatic exercises, individuals can experience a reduction in stress and an improvement in emotional regulation. This emotional balance is key to maintaining motivation and perseverance in the face of weight loss challenges. Furthermore, the practice promotes a positive and nurturing relationship with the body, which is essential for sustainable weight loss and self-care.

The integrative approach of somatic exercises aligns perfectly with the holistic perspective of this book. As we journey through the chapters, the connection between somatic practices, mindful eating, and nutritional insights will become increasingly clear. Each element of the book is designed to harmonize with the others, providing a comprehensive guide to physical and emotional well-being that supports weight loss in a healthy, sustainable manner.

In the subsequent sections, we will explore detailed somatic exercises, introduce mindful practices for emotional balance, and provide nutritional insights that together create a potent formula for weight loss and enhanced well-being. This book aims to empower readers to discover and embrace a lifestyle that balances physical health with emotional and mental wellness, guiding them toward a transformative journey of self-discovery and lasting change.

Somatic Exercises and Weight Loss

In health and fitness, weight loss is often a primary goal for many individuals. Yet, the journey to losing weight is not merely about the numbers on a scale; it encompasses a holistic approach that nurtures both your body and mind. This is where somatic exercises shine, offering a unique weight-loss pathway that transcends traditional exercise methods by fostering a deep, mindful connection with your body. In this section, we'll delve into how somatic exercises can be a powerful ally in achieving weight loss and enhancing overall well-being, seamlessly linking this concept with the comprehensive exploration of the book.

Somatic exercises, emphasizing mindful movement and body awareness, offer a nuanced approach to weight loss. Instead of focusing on high-intensity workouts that can often lead to burnout or injury, these practices encourage a gentle, sustainable path to physical health. By engaging in somatic exercises, you learn to listen to your body, recognizing signs of hunger, fullness, stress, and relaxation. This heightened awareness can lead to more mindful eating patterns and a reduction in stress-related eating, crucial factors in weight management.

Moreover, somatic exercises contribute to weight loss by improving metabolic function and body composition. As these exercises enhance flexibility, posture, and muscle tone, they also increase efficiency in movement. This improvement in physical functioning can boost metabolism, helping your body burn calories more effectively, even at rest. Additionally, the stress-reducing properties of somatic practices can lower levels of cortisol. This hormone contributes to weight gain, particularly in the abdominal area, and affects overall health negatively.

Beyond the physical aspects, somatic exercises offer profound emotional and mental health benefits that support weight loss journeys. Stress, anxiety, and negative body image can be significant barriers to weight loss. Through the mindful practice of somatic exercises, you can experience stress reduction and improve emotional regulation. This dynamic balance is key to maintaining motivation and perseverance in the face of weight loss challenges. Furthermore, the practice promotes a positive and nurturing relationship with your body, essential for sustainable weight loss and self-care.

The integrative approach of somatic exercises aligns perfectly with the holistic perspective of this book. As you journey through the chapters, the connection between somatic practices, mindful eating, and nutritional insights will become increasingly apparent. Each element of the book is designed to harmonize with the others, providing a comprehensive guide to physical and emotional well-being that supports weight loss in a healthy, sustainable manner.

In the subsequent sections, we will explore detailed somatic exercises, introduce mindful practices for emotional balance, and provide nutritional insights that together create a potent formula for weight loss and enhanced well-being. This book aims to empower you to discover and embrace a lifestyle that balances physical health with emotional and mental wellness, guiding you toward a transformative journey of self-discovery and lasting change.

Overview of the Book

Embark on a transformational journey with "Somatic Exercises for Beginners," a comprehensive guide that invites you to explore the harmonious blend of movement, mindfulness, and nutrition. This book is more than just a series of exercises; it is an invitation to delve into a holistic approach to health, promising physical enhancement and emotional and mental well-being. As you move through each chapter, you will be guided step-by-step, ensuring a deeply personal and engaging experience that resonates with your unique path toward health and happiness. Let's preview the enlightening voyage that awaits you within these pages.

In the Introduction to Somatic Exercises, we set the stage for what's to come, unveiling the rich tapestry of somatic practices. You'll discover the essence of somatics, learning how these exercises are not just physical movements but gateways to uniting body and mind. This foundational knowledge prepares you to engage with the transformative power somatics holds for your health and weight loss journey.

Chapter 1: Understanding Your Body encourages you to connect deeply with your physical self. You're empowered to tune into your body's signals through insights into body awareness, the impact of stress on weight, and emotional eating. This chapter is your first step toward holistic health, guiding you to listen and respond to your body's needs and signals.

Chapter 2: Foundations of Somatic Exercises dives into the principles that anchor somatic movements. Here, you're introduced to the critical elements of breath, posture, and alignment, equipping you with the knowledge to engage in somatic exercises effectively. This chapter is the cornerstone of your practice, ensuring you're well-prepared to embrace somatic movements' benefits fully.

Chapter 3: Somatic Exercises Explained transitions seamlessly from theory to action, offering a collection of bodily exercises with detailed guidance. Each movement is crafted to deepen your body awareness, alleviate discomfort, and enhance your connection to your body, making this chapter an indispensable, hands-on guide for your somatic journey.

Chapter 4: Mindful Practices for Emotional Balance widens the lens to include mindfulness, a crucial component in achieving emotional equilibrium. You'll explore practices that connect somatic exercises with mindful awareness, highlighting the powerful synergy between physical movement, mental health, and emotional well-being.

Chapter 5: Nutritional Insights for Weight Loss enriches your journey by integrating essential nutritional advice. This chapter aligns with the somatic and mindful practices you're learning, spotlighting foods that bolster energy, flexibility, and overall health, illustrating that true well-being extends beyond exercise to encompass the nourishment of the body.

Chapter 6: A 4-Week Somatic Exercise Plan for Beginners provides a concrete, day-by-day plan that blends exercises, mindfulness, and nutrition into a cohesive strategy for sustainable weight loss. This roadmap is your launchpad into a lifestyle where somatic practices are not just exercises but a way of life.

Chapter 7: Overcoming Challenges and Maintaining Progress tackles the hurdles and dips in motivation you may encounter. With strategies for overcoming obstacles, creating support systems, and sustaining motivation, this chapter gives you the tools to maintain your Progress and embrace long-term health.

"Somatic Exercises for Beginners" is not just a guide but a lifelong adventure in self-discovery and holistic health. The Conclusion ties together our journey, while Appendices offer additional resources and FAQs. Each chapter is designed to engage, educate, and empower you on your path to a healthier, more vibrant you. Welcome to your new beginning.

Chapter 1: Understanding Your Body

Welcome to the "Chapter 1: Understanding Your Body. Are you ready to explore your body and learn how it communicates with you? By becoming fluent in the language of your body, you'll gain insight and sensitivity to nourish, move, and love your body in ways that serve you best. Welcome to the transformation journey that begins with a single realization: to change your body, you must first understand it.

1.1 Body Awareness:

Imagine your body as a sophisticated instrument communicating through sensations, tension, relaxation, and movement. Body awareness is listening to this instrument's subtle cues, understanding its language, and responding appropriately to its needs. It's a foundational step that can profoundly change your weight loss journey and overall well-being.

Cultivating Mindful Movement

Start with mindful movement, a cornerstone of somatic exercises. Focus on the move as you engage in simple activities like walking or stretching. Notice how your joints articulate, how your weight shifts, and how your muscles engage. This practice helps to root you in the present moment, making you acutely aware of how your body moves and feels. It's not about exerting yourself but about observing and feeling the quality of movement.

Engaging in Body Scanning

Body scanning is another powerful technique for enhancing body awareness. Lie down in a comfortable position and mentally scan your body from head to toe. As you focus on each part, breathe into it, releasing tension and acknowledging any discomfort or ease you find. This practice increases awareness and begins releasing stress, setting a seamless transition to our next point, "The Science of Stress and Weight."

Exploring Proprioceptive Activities

Proprioception refers to the body's ability to sense its position and movements in space. Engaging in proprioceptive activities like balance exercises or closed-eye movements can sharpen your awareness and improve your connection to your body. Such practices train you to trust your body's signals, enhancing your ability to recognize when you're hungry, full, or simply eating out of stress.

Breathing for Awareness

Breath is life, and it's also a beacon for body awareness. By learning breathing techniques, you can notice the rhythm of your breath and how it affects your emotions and physical state. Deep abdominal breathing, for instance, can calm the nervous system and support a state of relaxation, making it easier for you to tap into a mindful state.

Integrating Daily Activities

Body awareness doesn't have to be limited to exercise. Integrate it into daily activities like eating. Chew slowly, savor the flavors, and notice how your body reacts to different foods. This can help prevent overeating and make meals more physically and emotionally satisfying.

By nurturing body awareness through these techniques, you'll become more attuned to your body's health and vitality needs. This awareness is your ally in recognizing the connection between stress and weight, which we'll explore in the next development point. Being mindful of your body's signals allows you to respond to them in ways that support weight loss and well-being instead of reacting unconsciously to habits or emotions.

Remember, this journey is about you. It's about transforming your relationship with your body and, by extension, with yourself. As you move through the exercises and techniques in this chapter, you'll lay the groundwork for a healthier, more balanced, and more connected life.

1.2 The Science of Stress and Weight:

You might wonder how an intangible feeling like stress can have a tangible impact on your weight. Stress, an inevitable part of life, sets off a cascade of hormonal reactions in your body. When you're stressed, your body releases adrenaline, which gives you an immediate energy boost, and cortisol, which tells your body to replenish that energy even if you haven't used many calories. This process served our ancestors well when their stress came from physical threats requiring energy. However, stress is often mental or emotional in today's world, and this fight-or-flight response can lead to weight gain.

Cortisol is particularly insidious in its effects on weight. It's known for encouraging fat storage, especially around the midsection, where it can be most harmful to health. Moreover, stress often disrupts sleep patterns, affecting metabolism and appetite-regulating hormones like ghrelin and leptin. You might reach for sugary snacks for a quick energy fix or crave carbohydrates because your body seeks instant energy to fuel your stress response.

But understanding the science of stress and weight is just the start. By recognizing how stress impacts your body, you're better prepared to counteract it. Somatic exercises, which you'll be introduced to in this book, are a potent antidote to stress. They encourage your body to shift from a state of tension and high alert to one of relaxation and recovery. Mindful practices like deep breathing and meditation can help stabilize cortisol levels and restore calm.

As we segue into "*1.3 Emotional Eating and How to Address It*", you'll see how the knowledge of stress's impact on weight is pivotal. Stress doesn't just lead to weight gain through hormonal changes; it also affects your behaviors, leading to emotional eating as a coping mechanism. You can break the cycle of stress and emotional eating by bringing somatic awareness and mindful practices into your eating habits. This isn't just about choosing a salad over a sandwich; it's about understanding why you make these choices and how you can make better ones by listening to your body's needs.

Remember, your journey with this book is about more than just weight loss. It's about equipping you with the understanding and tools to manage stress, engage with your body's signals, and make choices that enhance your overall well-being. As you learn to manage stress, you shed pounds and alleviate the burdens that weigh down your mind and spirit. This book is your guide through that journey, and as you turn each page, you'll find yourself equipped with more knowledge, practices, and insights that will help you lose weight and gain a more vibrant, healthful life.

1.3 Emotional Eating and How to Address It:

"Chapter 1: Understanding Your Body" highlights a hidden saboteur of wellness: emotional eating. This section guides you through the labyrinth of your cravings, where you will learn to identify the emotional factors that often lead you to the kitchen. This is not a battlefield of willpower but a dance of self-discovery. Emotional eating is a request from the body for comfort, not hunger. Here, you will get the tools to respond with heart, not habit.

Identifying Emotional Triggers
The first step to managing emotional eating is to identify your triggers. These could be stress, boredom, sadness, or even joy. You might reach for a snack when you're not physically hungry but emotionally seeking solace. Maintaining a food diary, you can effectively recognize the relationship between your food consumption and how it affects your physical and emotional well-being. Keeping a record of what you eat and drink and how you feel before and after consuming it can reveal patterns and help you make healthier choices. This will help you to see correlations between your emotions and food intake.

Strategies to Manage Emotional Eating
Once you've identified your triggers, it's time to develop strategies to cope with them. Let's look at a few:
- **Mindful Eating Practices:** Slow down and savor your food. Engage all your senses while eating and listen to your body's hunger and fullness cues. By practicing mindful eating, you can completely transform your relationship with food. You'll no longer be dependent on food to satisfy your emotions. Still, instead, you'll nourish your body and enjoy every bite. Give it a try and see how it changes your life!
- **Somatic Exercises:** These exercises can teach you to tune into your body's signals and emotions, helping you to distinguish between true hunger and emotional cravings. In "Chapter 2: Foundations of Somatic Exercises," you'll learn techniques that bring awareness and control to your physical state, which can be directly applied to managing emotional eating.
- **Stress Management Techniques:** Managing stress effectively can reduce the likelihood of emotional eating, a common trigger. Practices like deep breathing and yoga can be helpful relaxation and stress management techniques.
- **Alternative Coping Mechanisms**: Develop a toolkit of activities to turn to instead of food when emotions run high. This could be calling a friend, reading a book, or engaging in a hobby. The key is to find non-food ways to deal with emotions.
- **Nutritional Balance:** Sometimes, emotional eating can be triggered by a lack of certain nutrients. It is important to ensure that your diet is well-balanced and includes a variety of foods from different food groups.
- **Professional Support:** If emotional eating is deeply rooted, seeking the help of a professional such as a therapist or a dietitian can provide you with tailored strategies to overcome it.

As you progress through this chapter, you'll learn to identify and manage emotional eating and prepare to delve deeper into the world of somatic exercises in the next chapter. These exercises will offer a way to further connect with your body, understand its needs, and respond to emotions without relying on food. The journey you're on is holistic — it's about creating harmony between physical movement, emotional health, and nutrition to support a sustainable transformation.

Remember, addressing emotional eating isn't about perfection. It's about *progress, understanding, and developing a kinder relationship with yourself.* By implementing these strategies, you will have the tools to overcome emotional eating and confidently move forward. You'll take control of your life by what you eat and how you live it. You'll feel nourished, fulfilled, and empowered to make healthy choices.

Chapter 2: Foundations of Somatic Exercises

As you read "Chapter 2: Foundations of Somatic Exercises," immerse yourself in somatic movement principles. This section is the heart of somatic practice, where the dance of movement is less about the steps and more about the grace and awareness with which you perform them. Here, you'll learn the essence of mindfulness and internal focus. These fundamental principles are about moving and being moved from within.

2.1 Principles of Somatic Movement:
The Principle of Mindfulness
Mindfulness is the first beacon in the realm of somatic exercises. It's the art of being present in the moment, fully engaged with whatever you're doing. When you apply mindfulness to movement, each stretch and breath becomes an act of meditation. You can enhance your connection with your body by paying deliberate attention. This helps you notice even the slightest changes and subtle differences. Your body becomes like a vast landscape, where every hill and valley of muscle and tendon is a discovery waiting to be explored.

The Power of Internal Focus
Internal focus takes you deeper into the journey, guiding you to listen to the whispers of your body. It's about tuning into the dialogue between your muscles and your mind, feeling the interplay between tension and relaxation. This inward attention is transformative; it turns movement into a language through which your body communicates its stories, needs, and desires.

Integration with Breath
Your breath is your most faithful companion in somatic exercises. It's both the rhythm and the melody to which your body moves. As you'll discover in "2.2 Breathing Techniques," how you breathe can change how you move. Breath is not just a passive backdrop but an

active participant that shapes and informs every motion. It is the bridge between the mindful and the physical, carrying the weight of your attention into the fibers of your being.

The Dance of Control and Letting Go
Somatic movements are a delicate balance between control and surrender. You learn to control your movements to achieve precision and safety. Still, you're also invited to let go to allow the movements to flow naturally, without force or strain. This interplay creates a symphony of actions and reactions that teach you about the limits and capabilities of your body.

Embodied Learning
Somatic exercises are based on embodied learning, which involves learning by doing and feeling. You don't just execute movements; you experience them, and through that experience, you gain knowledge. This knowledge isn't abstract; it's felt, it's lived. It's the knowing that changes not just how you move but how you think and feel.

The Continuum of Movement
Finally, you'll understand that somatic movement is not a static practice but a continuum. There is no 'perfect' way to move, only the perfect one for you now. Your training and understanding of these principles will evolve as you do.

As you explore the basic principles of somatic movement, let them guide your exercises and influence your life. Embrace mindfulness, internal focus, and intentional breathing as your companions beyond the yoga mat. Carry these principles with you into "2.2 Breathing Techniques" and allow them to be the foundation that integrates your physical, emotional, and nutritional well-being into a cohesive whole. This chapter is more than just a set of instructions; it's an invitation to engage in a deeper and more intimate dialogue with your body.

2.2 Breathing Techniques:

This section is your guide to harnessing *the power of your breath* — a vital force that nourishes your body with every inhale and releases tension with every exhale.

Breath is your body's intrinsic rhythm, and learning to master it is akin to a musician fine-tuning an instrument. Through breathing techniques, you'll cultivate a serenity that permeates not just moments of stillness but also weaves through the fabric of your daily life. Let's explore how controlled breathing can become a sanctuary for relaxation and a fortress against stress.

Diaphragmatic Breathing: The Foundation
Begin with diaphragmatic breathing, the cornerstone of respiratory exercises. As you breathe deeply, your diaphragm — that muscular partition beneath your lungs — engages, providing your body with a more profound oxygen exchange. This type of breathing encourages a relaxation response in the body, countering the effects of stress and calming the mind. You'll learn to feel the expansion of your lungs and the gentle rise and fall of your abdomen as a physical affirmation of tranquility.

Rhythmic Breathing: The Flow
Next, you'll move into rhythmic breathing, where the goal is to create a steady flow of breath that becomes a meditative cadence. This practice helps regulate your emotional state and anchors you in the present moment, creating a bridge between the conscious and the subconscious mind. You'll cultivate a sense of balance and peace that helps dissolve stress as you synchronize your breath with your movements, preparing your body and mind for the upcoming exercises.

4-7-8 Breathing: The Relaxation Breath
The 4-7-8 technique is a simple yet powerful method to instill a sense of calm quickly. By inhaling for four counts, holding for seven, and exhaling for eight, you activate your parasympathetic nervous system — the part of your body responsible for rest and digestion. This technique is beneficial when stress levels rise or

sleep seems elusive, making it a valuable tool in your relaxation repertoire.

Alternate Nostril Breathing: The Balancer
Alternate nostril breathing is a practice borrowed from ancient yogic traditions, known for its ability to harmonize the left and right hemispheres of the brain. It's a practice of balance, ideal for those moments when stress has tilted your inner equilibrium. By alternately breathing through one nostril at a time, you'll create a sense of peace and focus that sets the stage for mindful posture and movement.

Breathing with Movement: The Integration
As you'll discover in "2.3 Posture and Alignment," breathing is not just a solitary practice but an integral part of all somatic exercises. You'll learn to integrate breathing into your movements, enhancing the effectiveness of each pose and sequence. The breath will guide you into deeper stretches, support you in maintaining challenging postures, and assist in releasing tension from the body.

By mastering these breathing techniques, you're learning to relax and transform your breath into a tool for profound change. Each inhale brings vitality and awareness; each exhale releases old patterns and stress. This section isn't just about breathing; it's about relearning how to live quickly and gracefully. As you carry these practices with you, they'll become a natural part of your daily routine, paving the way for a life with more presence, calm, and well-being.

2.3 Posture and Alignment:
You have now reached the section about Posture and Alignment. This section focuses on the natural stance and structure of your body, which is a crucial element in the practice of somatic exercises and plays a fundamental role in promoting your overall well-being. In the previous section, you learned to tune into the rhythm of your breath. Now, you can move on to the next step.

Imagine posture and alignment as the foundation on which your body is constructed. Just as a building relies on a solid foundation to maintain its integrity, your body depends on proper posture and alignment to function optimally. In the context of somatic exercises, these principles are not about rigid standards or aesthetic ideals but about finding the natural equilibrium that allows your body to move with efficiency and grace.

The Pillars of Posture
Posture is more than standing up straight—it's an ongoing dialogue between your body and gravity. Good posture distributes the forces of gravity evenly across your body, minimizing strain and maximizing support. When you stand, sit, or move with proper alignment, you are poised to engage in somatic exercises with a reduced risk of injury and an increased capacity for adequate movement.

Alignment: The Blueprint of Movement
Alignment refers to how the head, shoulders, spine, hips, knees, and ankles relate and line up with each other. Proper alignment is crucial because it ensures that your muscles, joints, and ligaments work together harmoniously. This blueprint guides each movement in somatic practice, ensuring each action is as beneficial as possible.

The Role of Alignment in Somatic Practice
In somatic exercises, where the goal is to cultivate a deeper awareness and connection with your body, alignment is not merely physical—it's also a state of attunement. Each exercise in somatic practice is an opportunity to refine your alignment. As you progress into "Chapter 3: Somatic Exercises Explained," you'll understand how each movement expresses balance and poise.

Somatics: A Mirror for Posture
Somatic exercises act as a mirror, reflecting the state of your body's posture and alignment. You can identify areas of tension and misalignment through slow, mindful movements. These

exercises then become a path to re-educating your body, teaching it to let go of habitual patterns that disrupt balance and to embrace a new way of moving that supports structural integrity.

The Interplay of Breath and Posture

Breathing, which you've explored in depth, intertwines with posture and alignment. Breathing deeply can enhance your posture; conversely, a well-aligned body allows for more efficient breathing. This reciprocal relationship is a golden thread that runs through the tapestry of somatic practices.

From Awareness to Practice

As you transition into the practical applications in the next chapter, remember that posture and alignment are not static but dynamic aspects of your being. They change and adapt as you move and breathe. The somatic exercises you're about to learn are not just movements to be performed; they are expressions of the living art of posture and alignment.

By understanding and applying the principles of posture and alignment, you set the stage for a somatic practice that is both safe and effective. You prepare your body to engage in each movement with clarity and precision, laying the groundwork for a deeper exploration of somatic exercises that enhance your physical and emotional well-being and support your journey toward harmonious living.

Chapter 3: Somatic Exercises Explained

Now, we embark on a journey to transform your movement and awareness. In this section, you will begin a conversation between your body and mind, becoming more in tune with the subtle workings of your being. These initial movements are not just precursors to the practice but intentional acts that awaken the senses and prepare the muscles for the more prosperous and complex sequences that will follow.

With the warm-up movements, you will awaken each muscle group, preparing your body.

Consider this warm-up an essential ritual, a time to honor the vessel that carries you and set an intention for future practice. With each breath and movement, you are preparing your body and opening the door to a deeper connection with yourself.

Before diving into these exercises, ensure you have the necessary materials to support your journey. A yoga mat for a comfortable, non-slip surface. Comfortable clothing allows unrestricted movement, and props like foam rollers or yoga blocks can support and deepen the stretches. Remember also to keep a water bottle handy to stay hydrated, and consider keeping a blanket nearby for exercises done in a sitting or lying position.

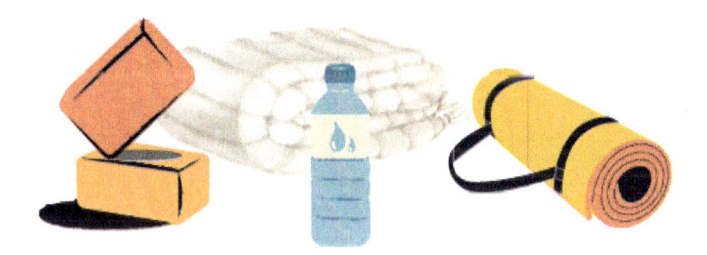

Before you start with the exercises, here are a few tips to follow to get into your practice:

Think of warm-up movements as a gentle awakening. With each motion, you're coaxing your body out of stillness and into a state of readiness. It's a process of gradually increasing your heart rate, warming up your muscles, and signaling to your nervous system that it's time to move. This approach respects your body's natural pace, allowing you to ease into activity without shock or strain.

Experience the power of flow and fluidity with these warm-up exercises. Allow your body to move easily and gracefully as you engage in smooth, continuous movements that align with your natural rhythms. Incorporating these simple yet effective exercises into your routine will help you prepare your body and mind for any physical activity, allowing you to perform at your best. Get started today and feel the difference in your body's agility and flexibility! Imagine your arms are like branches swaying in a gentle breeze, your spine like a stream of water flowing over smooth rocks. This visualization helps to dissolve any stiffness and cultivate a state of suppleness and ease.

As you begin these warm-up movements, **bring the mindfulness you've cultivated from the earlier chapters to the forefront**. Stay fully present with the sensations that arise with each stretch and bend. Note the warmth spreading through your muscles, the subtle release of tension, and the dialogue of comfort and challenge. Here, mindfulness transforms your warm-up from routine to revelation.

Let your breath be your guide. Coordinate your movements with your inhales and exhales, allowing the rhythm of your breathing to set the pace. This harmonization enhances the warm-up's efficacy and deepens your connection to the exercise, ensuring your body and breath move.

These initial movements prepare for the more focused work in "3.2 Core Somatic Movements". They establish a foundation of warmth and awareness to support the more intensive exercises. When you transition to the core movements, your body will be more receptive, responsive, and engaged, ready to delve into the somatic experience with its entire presence.

Remember, your warm-up movements also reflect the nutritional insights you've learned. Just as you nourish your body with wholesome foods to prepare for the day, these movements nourish your body with energy and awareness to prepare for more intensive somatic work. Each motion feeds your body with vitality, just as each healthy meal fuels your journey toward well-being.

Embrace these warm-up exercises as an essential part of your practice, a dedicated time to honor your body's needs and to set the stage for deeper exploration. This is where you begin to translate the principles of somatic movement into action, where you step into the flow of your progress, and prepare yourself for the transformative work to come.

3.1 Warm-Up Movements
Neck Tilts

This warm-up exercise targets the neck muscles, promoting flexibility and tension release. To perform neck tilts correctly, follow these steps:

1. **Starting Position**: Sit or stand with your spine in a neutral position, shoulders relaxed and down away from your ears, and your eyes looking straight ahead.
2. **Initial Movement**: Begin by gently lowering your right ear towards your right shoulder, keeping your left shoulder relaxed and stationary. Avoid raising your shoulder to meet your ear; the movement should come solely from your neck.
3. **Hold and Feel**: Hold this position for a few seconds, feeling a gentle stretch along the left side of your neck. The stretch should be comfortable and soothing, not painful.
4. **Return to Center**: Slowly bring your head back to the neutral starting position, realigning your neck and head with your spine.
5. **Repeat on Opposite Side**: Now, gently lower your left ear towards your left shoulder, ensuring your right shoulder stays relaxed and doesn't creep up.

6. **Hold and Breathe**: Again, hold for a moment, taking deep breaths to help deepen the stretch on the right side of your neck
7. **Frequency**: Alternate these tilts gently from side to side, moving slowly and with control. Perform this tilt 5-10 times for each side.

During neck tilts, **maintain mindfulness** about the rest of your body. Keep the rest of your posture stable and your face relaxed. The movement should not be forced but rather a natural inclination that allows the neck muscles to elongate and relax.

Remember, the key to this warm-up is gentleness. The neck is a sensitive area, and overstretching can lead to strain. As you become more familiar with your range of motion, you can gradually increase the depth of the tilt, always listening to your body's feedback. This exercise warms the neck muscles and increases proprioceptive awareness, which is critical for all subsequent somatic practices.

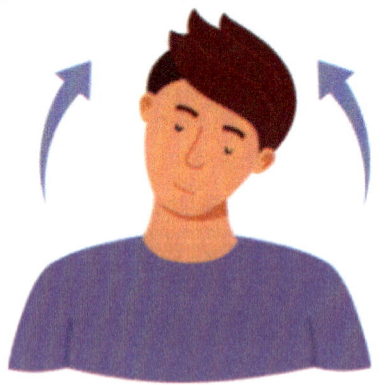

Neck Tilts

Shoulder Rolls

This warm-up exercise is excellent for relieving stiffness and increasing mobility in the shoulder joints, which is very useful if you spend many hours sitting in front of the computer, for example. Here's how to perform shoulder rolls with attention to detail:

1. **Starting Position**: Stand or sit up straight with your feet hip-width apart if standing. Let your arms hang naturally at your sides. Keep your neck relaxed and gaze forward.
2. **Upward Phase**: Inhale and lift your shoulders straight up towards your ears. This upward movement is deliberating, engaging the upper trapezius muscles.
3. **Backward Phase**: Exhale and gently roll your shoulders back, drawing big circles with them. Imagine you're trying to touch your shoulder blades together. This motion opens up the chest and engages the upper back muscles.
4. **Downward Phase**: Continue rolling by bringing the shoulders down, feeling the shoulder blades slide down your back. This helps to stretch and release any accumulated tension in the shoulder area.
5. **Forward Phase**: Complete the circle by rolling your shoulders forward and rounding the upper back slightly. You'll feel a slight contraction in the chest and front of the shoulders.
6. **Coordinate your breath** with the movement, inhaling as the shoulders go up and exhaling as they roll back and down. This coordination enhances the relaxation effect of the exercise.
7. **Repetition**: Perform this rolling action slowly for about 30 seconds to a minute, or about 8-10 full rolls.
8. **Reverse Direction**: After completing the rolls in one direction, reverse the movement, up, back, and down. This ensures that the muscles and joints are warmed up evenly.
9. **Mindfulness**: As you perform this exercise, focus on the sensation in your shoulders. Pay attention to any areas of tightness or discomfort, using the movement to work through and release those sensations gently.

Remember that each movement in somatic practice is an opportunity for increased body awareness. As you roll your shoulders, be aware of how the movement affects your posture and sensations in the upper body.

Shoulder rolls prepare the muscles for more intensive somatic work and contribute to better posture and alignment, which will be vital as you move into "Core Somatic Movements" and beyond. Through regular practice, you'll increase the range of motion in your shoulders and encourage relaxation throughout your upper body.

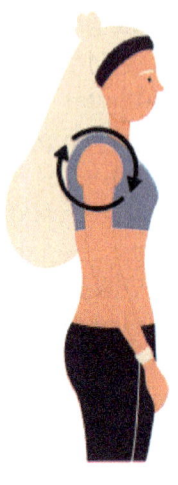

Shoulder rolls

<u>Arm Circles</u>

This dynamic warm-up exercise is designed to engage and enhance the flexibility and mobility of your shoulder joints and the surrounding muscles. Properly executed arm circles warm up the deltoids, trapezius, rotator cuff group, and pectorals. Here's a detailed guide to performing arm circles:

1. **Starting Position**: Stand with your feet shoulder-width apart to maintain balance. Extend your arms straight out to the sides so they are parallel to the floor, palms facing down.
2. **Small Circles Forward**: Begin by making small, controlled circular motions with your arms moving forward. Concentrate on engaging the muscles around your shoulders. Keep the circles tight and precise.
3. **Gradual Increase in Size**: Gradually increase the diameter of your circles, allowing your shoulder joints to warm up

and increase their range of motion. Ensure that these larger circles are still controlled and smooth.
4. **Maintain Posture**: As you perform the arm circles, keep your posture erect, your core engaged, and your spine neutral. Avoid arching your back or swaying your body, which could compromise the effectiveness of the warm-up and lead to potential strain.
5. **Breathing**: Coordinate your breathing by inhaling deeply as your arms go up and exhaling as they come down. This rhythmic breathing will help oxygenate your muscles and keep you centered and focused.
6. **Reverse Direction**: After completing the forward circles for about 30 seconds, reverse the direction. Now, perform the backward circles, starting with small and widening circles. This ensures balanced muscle activation on both the anterior and posterior sides of the body.
7. **Large Circles**: Once adequately warmed up with smaller circles, you can perform extensive, slow processes to maximize the shoulder joint's range of motion. Keep the movement controlled, focusing on the sensation of the muscles stretching and warming.
8. **Soft Knees**: Keep a slight bend in your knees throughout the exercise to prevent any unnecessary strain on your lower back and to maintain a stable base.
9. **Gaze and Neck Position**: Maintain a relaxed gaze forward, ensuring your neck is not strained as your arms circle. The neck should remain in a neutral position.
10. **Frequency and Duration**: Continue with the arm circles for a duration that feels sufficient for your body, generally between 30 seconds to a minute in each direction. Listen to your body, and let your muscles' response to the movement dictate the duration.

Arm circles are a fundamental warm-up exercise that helps transition your body from rest to active engagement.

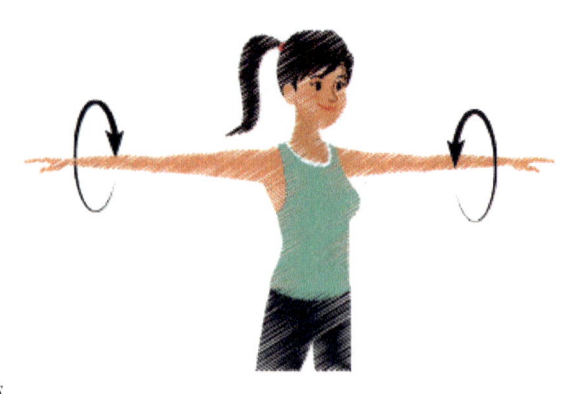

Arm Circles

Wrist Loosening

This warm-up exercise is perfect for increasing mobility and flexibility in the wrists, essential for activities requiring hand strength and precision. This movement helps prevent strain and injuries by preparing the wrist joints for more demanding tasks. Here's how to perform wrist-loosening exercises with attention to detail:

1. **Starting Position**: Begin by extending your arms in front of you at shoulder height, keeping them straight. Your palms can face down to start. Ensure your shoulders are relaxed and down, away from your ears, to maintain a neutral spine.
2. **Initial Rotation**: Start rotating your wrists slowly in a clockwise direction. Focus on making the movement as smooth and controlled as possible, exploring the full range of motion without causing discomfort. The movement should originate from the wrists, keeping the rest of the arm stationary.
3. **Reverse Direction**: After completing several rotations in a clockwise direction, pause briefly and then switch to rotate your wrists counterclockwise. This ensures balanced mobility work on both sides of each wrist.
4. **Mindful Breathing**: Inhale deeply as you begin the rotation, and exhale as you complete each circle. This

synchronization of breath with movement enhances focus and relaxation.
5. **Alternate Hand Positions**: To comprehensively warm up the wrists, alternate your hand positions. After doing rotations with palms facing down, flip your hands so your palms face up and repeat the rotations in both directions. This variation ensures all the muscles and tendons around the wrists are adequately warmed up.
6. **Flexion and Extension**: Add wrist flexion and extension movements by holding your arm out, palm facing down, and gently pulling the fingers back towards you with the other hand to stretch the underside of the wrist. Then, point your fingers down and gently apply pressure to stretch the top of the wrist. These movements complement the rotations by stretching the wrists in all directions.
7. **Frequency and Duration**: Perform wrist rotations for 30 seconds to 1 minute in each direction. The goal is to feel the joints lubricating and the muscles around the wrists warming up without pushing into pain.
8. **Awareness and Adjustment** - Pay attention to how your wrists feel during the exercise. Adjust the intensity or range of motion if you encounter any stiffness or discomfort. The objective is gentle mobilization, not strain.
9.

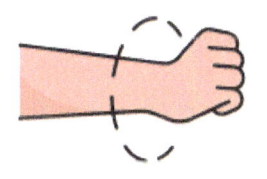

Wrist Loosening

Side Stretches

This warm-up exercise is essential for lengthening and loosening the lateral muscles of the body, including the obliques and intercostal muscles. Side stretches enhance flexibility, improve posture, and increase the range of motion in your spine and torso, preparing you for activities that require bending, twisting, or extensive arm movements. Here's a detailed breakdown of how to perform side stretches effectively:

1. **Starting Position**: Stand with your feet hip-width apart to ensure a stable base. Keep your knees slightly bent to protect your lower back, and engage your core muscles to support your spine.
2. **Initial Stretch**: Extend your right arm straight above your head, keeping your elbow close to your ear. Ensure your shoulder does not creep up to your ear but stays relaxed and down to maximize the stretch along your side.
3. **Engage the Stretch**: While keeping your feet firmly planted and your hips facing forward, gently bend your torso to the left side. The movement should originate from your waist, allowing the stretch to extend through the side of your body. Keep your left hand on your hip or extend it down the side of your leg to maintain balance and enhance the stretch.
4. **Breath and Depth**: Inhale as you reach upwards, exhale as you extend into the bend, deepening the stretch. Use your breath to guide the movement, allowing each exhale to take you deeper into the stretch without forcing it.
5. **Hold and Focus**: Hold the stretch for 20 to 30 seconds, focusing on lengthening the side of your body with each breath. You should feel a continuous, gentle pull along the outside of your torso, from your hip to your fingertips.
6. **Return to Center**: Slowly bring your torso back upright, lowering your right arm. Take a moment to notice the sensations in your body before repeating the stretch on the opposite side.
7. **Repeat on Opposite Side**: Extend your left arm above your head and gently bend to the right, following the same steps to ensure both sides of your body are equally stretched and warmed up.
8. **Mindfulness and Alignment**: Throughout the exercise, maintain mindfulness of your body's alignment. Ensure your bend is directly to the side rather than forward or

backward to effectively isolate and stretch the lateral muscles.
9. **Modifications and Variations**: For more profound engagement, you can perform this stretch while seated on the floor with your legs crossed. This can help stabilize the hips and isolate the stretch in the upper body. Alternatively, holding a lightweight or a yoga block in the extended hand can increase the intensity of the stretch for those seeking a deeper warm-up.

Side stretches are essential for warming up before exercise and countering the effects of sitting or standing for long periods. Incorporating them into your routine will improve your flexibility and movement efficiency and prepare your body for more dynamic movements.

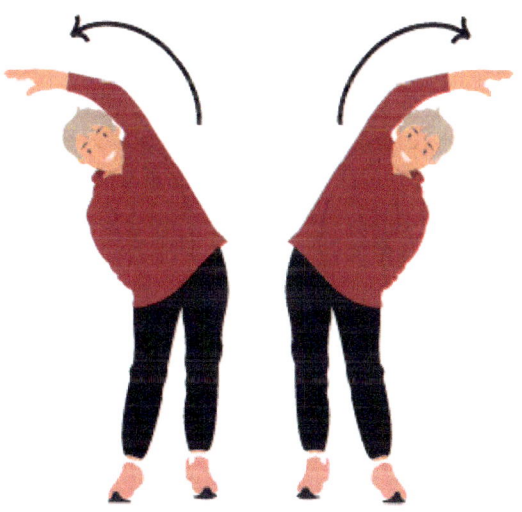

Side Stretches

<u>Spinal Twists</u>

This versatile warm-up exercise is pivotal for enhancing spinal mobility, relieving tension in the back, and promoting overall flexibility. Spinal twists target the muscles surrounding the spine, including the erector spine, obliques, and transverse abdominis, and gently massage the internal organs, improving digestive health. Whether performed sitting or standing, spinal twists help prepare your body for various movements and activities. Here's how to execute spinal twists with precision and care:

1. **Starting Position (Standing)**: Stand with your feet shoulder-width apart knees slightly bent to maintain flexibility in the lower body. Your arms can be extended to the sides at shoulder height or placed on your hips.
2. **Starting Position (Sitting)**: Sit on the edge of a sturdy chair or floor with your legs crossed, your spine tall, and your shoulders relaxed. Ensure your sitting bones are evenly grounded to support an upright posture.
3. **Initiate the Twist (Standing)**: Begin by slowly turning your torso to the right, keeping your hips facing forward to isolate the rotation in the upper body. Allow your head to follow the movement of your torso so your neck remains in alignment with your spine.
4. **Initiate the Twist (Sitting)**: Place your right hand on your left knee and your left hand behind your back or on the seat for support. Gently twist your torso to the left, leading with your shoulders and allowing your head to turn last.
5. **Breathing and Deepening**: Inhale deeply in the starting position, and as you exhale, deepen into the twist. Focus on lengthening your spine with each inhalation and rotating further with each exhalation without forcing the movement.
6. **Hold and Focus**: Hold the twist for 20 to 30 seconds, concentrating on the sensation of stretching and opening across your torso and back. Maintain even deep breaths to help facilitate relaxation and mobility in the twist.
7. **Return to Center**: Inhale as you slowly unwind your torso, returning to the center. Pause momentarily to notice any sensations in your spine and back before twisting to the opposite side.
8. **Repeat on the Opposite Side**: Perform the twist on the opposite side, ensuring that you spend equal time and effort on both sides to promote symmetrical spinal mobility.

9. **Mindfulness and Alignment**: Focus on keeping your movements slow and controlled throughout the exercise. Please pay special attention to your spine, imagining it lengthening upwards as you twist to avoid compression.
10. **Modifications and Variations**: For an added stretch, the standing version can include reaching the opposite hand to the outside of the leg or using a wall for resistance. In the sitting version, varying the position of your hands can intensify or lessen the stretch, depending on your comfort and flexibility.

Spinal twists lubricate the vertebral discs, increase circulation in the back, and promote body awareness and fluidity in movement. Incorporating spinal twists in your warm-up routine can enhance your spine's health and mobility in the long run.

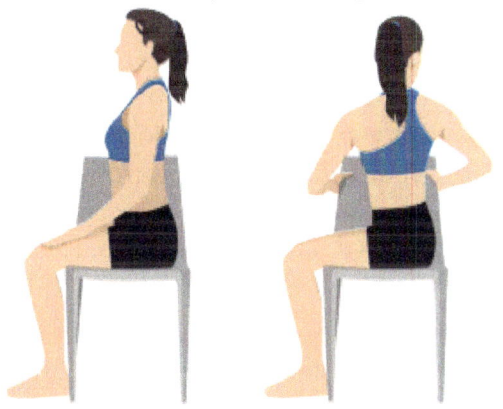

Spinal Twists

<u>Cat-Cow Stretches</u>

This fundamental warm-up exercise is revered for its ability to increase spinal flexibility, enhance breath coordination, and gently tone the core. By alternating between arching the back and dipping it downward, Cat-Cow stretches stimulate the spinal column, relieve tension in the back muscles, and promote a fluid connection between movement and breath. Here's how to perform Cat-Cow stretches with attention to detail and mindfulness:

1. **Starting Position**: Begin on your hands and knees on a comfortable, stable surface like a yoga mat. Position your wrists directly under your shoulders and your knees under your hips. Spread your fingers wide for a stable base, and ensure your spine is in a neutral position, with your head in line with your spine, gazing down at the floor. You can do it in a chair if you have trouble with the quadrupedal position.
2. **Cat Pose**: Inhale to prepare. As you exhale, initiate the movement by rounding your spine upwards towards the ceiling like a cat stretching. Tuck your chin towards your chest, allowing your neck to relax. Engage your abdominal muscles to support the spine as it arches, pushing the floor away with your hands and knees. Imagine drawing your belly button up towards your spine to deepen the arch.
3. **Transition**: Pause at the top of the arch, taking a moment to feel the stretch along your spine.
4. **Cow Pose**: On your next inhalation, reverse the movement by allowing your belly to sink towards the floor, lifting your sit bones and chest towards the ceiling. Your back will naturally dip down. Lift your head to look straight ahead or slightly upward, but be careful not to strain the neck. This position encourages a gentle stretch across your abdomen and chest, promoting flexibility in the spine's lumbar and cervical regions.
5. **Breathing and Movement Coordination**: The fluid movement between Cat and Cow should be synchronized with your breath. Exhale as you round the spine into Cat pose, and inhale as you soften into Cow pose. This coordination enhances the massage effect on the spine and encourages a deep connection between breath and movement.
6. **Repetition**: Flow between Cat and Cow poses for 1-2 minutes, allowing the rhythm of your breath to guide the pace of the exercise. Focus on the sensation of each

vertebra moving, promoting mobility and flexibility throughout the entire spine.
7. **Mindfulness and Observation**: As you move through Cat-Cow stretches, remain mindful of the sensations in your body. Notice areas of tension and ease, using the movement to explore and gently release any stiffness in the back.
8. **Modifications and Variations**: Cat-Cow can be modified for those with wrist discomfort by coming onto the fists or using yoga blocks under the hands.

Cat-Cow stretches ready the spine for movement and aligns the breath and mind with the body, creating a foundation of awareness and presence that supports the entire somatic journey.

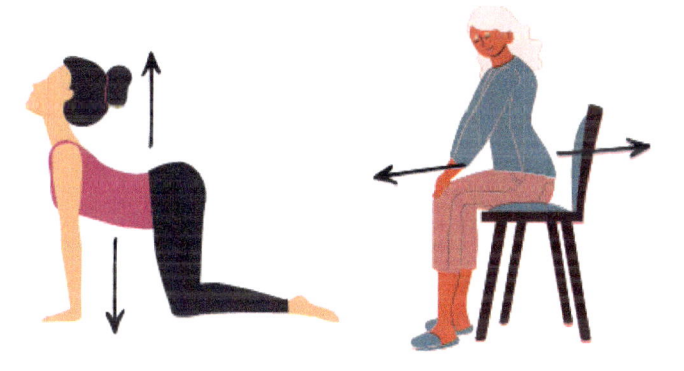

Cat-Cow Stretches

Pelvic Tilts

This warm-up exercise can help alleviate lower back discomfort, improve posture, and form the foundation for core stability. Here's a detailed guide to performing pelvic tilts correctly:
1. **Starting Position**: Lie on your back on a comfortable, flat surface like a yoga mat. Bend your knees, keeping your feet flat on the floor about hip-width apart. Place your arms by

your sides with palms facing down. Ensure your spine is in a neutral position with its natural curves.
2. **Find Neutral Pelvis**: Find a neutral pelvis position before initiating the movement. This means your pubic bone and hip bones should be on the same plane, neither tilting forward nor backward. You can place your hands on your hips to feel this alignment.
3. **Initiate the Tilt (Posterior Tilt)**: Exhale and gently engage your abdominal muscles to tilt your pelvis towards your face. This action will flatten your lower back against the floor. Think of it as gently scooping your pelvis upward. The movement is small and controlled, originating from the lower abdominals and the pelvis, not the legs or glutes.
4. **Return to Neutral**: Inhale and slowly release the tilt, allowing your pelvis to return to the neutral position. Pay attention to the movement, ensuring a smooth transition back to the starting alignment.
5. **Initiate the Tilt (Anterior Tilt)**: On your next inhale, gently arch your lower back by tilting your pelvis away from your face. This introduces a slight gap between your lower back and the floor, engaging your muscles.
6. **Breathing and Movement Coordination**: Coordinate your breath with the movement – exhaling as you tilt the pelvis upward (posterior tilt) and inhaling as you return to neutral or tilt downwards (anterior tilt). This coordination enhances the effectiveness of the exercise and maintains a rhythm that supports mindful movement.
7. **Repetition**: Rock your pelvis back and forth between the posterior and anterior tilts for about 1-2 minutes. Focus on the sensation of the movement and the gentle engagement of your core and lower back muscles.
8. **Mindfulness and Focus**: Maintain a focus on the pelvic region throughout the exercise. Visualize the movement, which helps lubricate the joints and gently stretch the lower back muscles. It's a subtle motion that requires concentration to perform correctly.

9. **Modifications and Variations**: For added engagement, you can lift your feet off the floor, bringing your knees directly above your hips, and perform the tilts in this position. This variation increases the challenge to your abdominal muscles.

As you progress through your somatic practice, the awareness and control gained from pelvic tilts will support more complex exercises and movements, ensuring a solid foundation for physical health and well-being.

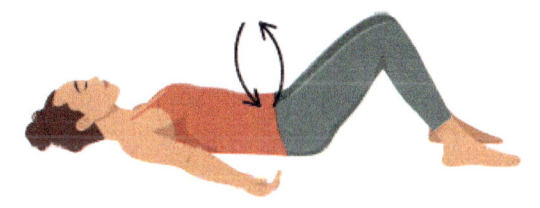

Pelvic Tilts

<u>Hip Circles</u>

This dynamic warm-up exercise focuses on mobilizing the hip joints, enhancing flexibility, and increasing blood flow to the surrounding muscles. Hip circles are particularly beneficial for those who experience stiffness due to prolonged sitting or wish to improve their range of motion for athletic performance. By engaging in this exercise, you prepare your body for more complex movements, ensuring the hips are loose and warmed up. Here's a step-by-step guide to performing hip circles effectively:

1. **Starting Position**: Stand with your feet shoulder-width apart, ensuring stable footing. Place your hands on your hips or extend them outward for balance. Keep your spine long and your shoulders relaxed, establishing a posture that promotes free movement of the hips.
2. **Initiate the Movement**: Begin the exercise by pushing your hips forward slightly, engaging the muscles in your lower back and abdominals. This forward motion is the starting point of your circle.

3. **Move to the Side**: Continue the circular motion by moving your hips to the right, engaging the side muscles, and stretching the opposite leg's inner thigh. Keep your upper body as stationary as possible, isolating the movement to the hips.
4. **Push Backwards**: From the side position, push your hips backward, engaging your glutes and stretching the front hip flexors. This part of the circle helps counteract the effects of sitting by opening up the front of the hips.
5. **Complete the Circle**: Continue moving your hips to the left, balancing the stretch and mobilization on both sides of your body. Finish the circle by returning to the starting position with your hips pushed slightly forward.
6. **Reverse Direction**: After completing several circles in one direction, reverse the movement to ensure balanced hip mobility. Start by pushing your hips forward, then to the left, backward, and right, completing the circle in the opposite direction.
7. **Breathing and Movement Coordination**: Coordinate your breathing with the movement, inhaling as you move your hips forward and to the side and exhaling as you push your hips back and complete the circle. This coordination helps deepen the exercise's effectiveness and maintain a rhythmic flow.
8. **Repetition**: Perform the hip circles for about 1-2 minutes, alternating directions every few circles. Focus on the smoothness and fluidity of the movement, gradually increasing the range of motion as your hips loosen up.
9. **Mindfulness and Focus**: Pay close attention to the sensations in your hip joints and surrounding muscles. Notice areas of tightness or ease, using the exercise to explore and release tension.
10. **Modification and variations:** For an added challenge, you can perform hip circles while standing on one leg, which introduces a balance component and engages

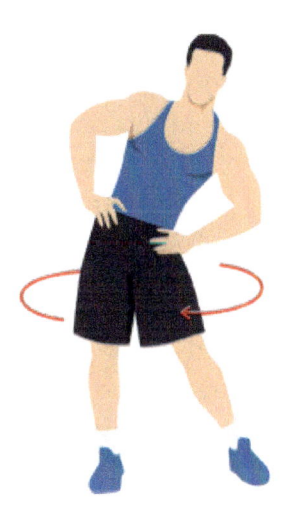

Hip circles

__Knee Hugs__

This warm-up exercise targets the lower back, hips, and hamstrings, offering a simple yet effective way to release tension. By gently pulling the knee towards the chest, you stretch to alleviate tightness, enhance mobility, and prepare the body for more dynamic movements. Knee hugs are a therapeutic movement for those experiencing lower back discomfort. Here's a detailed guide to performing knee hugs properly:
1. **Starting Position**: Lie flat on your back on a comfortable, supportive surface like a yoga mat. Keep your legs extended and your arms by your sides. Ensure your spine is neutral, with your lower back slightly touching the mat.
2. **Initiate the Stretch**: Bend your right knee and bring it towards your chest. Wrap your hands around your shin or the back of your thigh, whichever is more comfortable and accessible, avoiding any strain on the knee.
3. **Deepen the Stretch**: Pull your right knee closer to your chest, using your hands to apply light pressure. Keep your left leg straight and grounded on the mat, or for a modified

stretch, bend the left knee with the foot flat on the floor to reduce strain on the lower back.
4. **Hold and Breathe**: Hold this position for 20 to 30 seconds, focusing on relaxing your lower back and hips with each exhale. You should feel a gentle stretch in your right glute, hip, and lower back. Avoid jerking or forceful pulling; the movement should be smooth and controlled.
5. **Release and Repeat**: Slowly return your right leg to the starting position. Pause for a moment to notice any sensations in your lower back and right hip. Then, repeat the stretch with your left knee, ensuring equal treatment on both sides to maintain balance in flexibility and muscle relaxation.
6. **Breathing and Movement Coordination**: Coordinate your breath with the movement by inhaling as you prepare to lift your knee and exhaling as you pull it closer to your chest. This rhythmic breathing facilitates relaxation and can help deepen the stretch gently.
7. **Mindfulness and Observation**: Remember the sensations in your lower back and hips as you perform the knee hugs. Use this time to connect with your body, noticing areas of tension or ease. The goal is to nurture your body through the stretch, not to push it to discomfort.
8. **Modifications and Variations**: For an added stretch, gently rock side to side while hugging your knee to massage your lower back on the mat. Alternatively, you can simultaneously bring both knees to your chest for a more intense stretch in the lower back and hips.

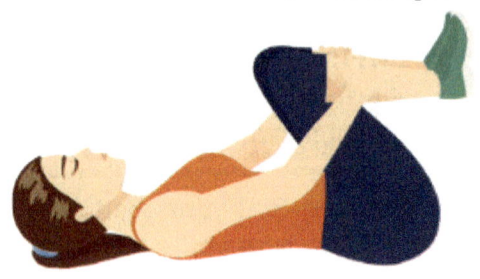

Knee Hugs

Leg Swings

This warm-up exercise prepares your legs for a wide range of activities by increasing flexibility, improving range of motion, and stimulating blood flow to the lower body. Leg swings target the hips, hamstrings, quadriceps, and groin area, making them an excellent choice for athletes, dancers, or anyone looking to enhance their lower body mobility. Here's a detailed breakdown of how to perform leg swings correctly:

- **Starting Position**: Find a stable support, such as a wall, chair, or ballet barre. Stand upright and face the support, placing one hand on it for balance. Keep your weight lightly on your supporting leg, which should slightly bend to absorb movement.

Forward and Backward Swings:
1. **Initiate the Swing**: Shift your weight to your supporting leg. Begin with the portion you intend to swing first, keeping it straight but not locked at the knee.
2. **Forward Swing**: Gently swing the leg forward, raising it as comfortably as possible without bending at the waist. Aim for a smooth, controlled motion, engaging your core for stability.

Backward Swing:

3. After reaching the peak of the forward swing, let momentum carry your leg back through the starting position and behind you. Keep your torso upright and avoid arching your back excessively as the leg swings backward.
4. **Breathing**: Inhale as you swing the leg forward and exhale as you swing it back. Proper breathing helps maintain rhythm and balance throughout the exercise.
5. **Repetition**: Perform 10-15 swings on one leg, then switch to the other, ensuring both sides are equally warmed up.

Side-to-Side Swings:

6. **Position Adjustment**: Turn to stand perpendicular to your support, holding it with the hand closest to it for balance.
7. **Initiate the Swing**: Start with your closest leg to the support and swing it out to the side, away from your body.
8. **Side Swing**: Lift your leg sideways as comfortably as possible, focusing on engaging the muscles on the outer thigh and hip.
9. **Crossing Swing**: After reaching the peak of the side swing, cross the leg in front of your supporting leg, engaging the inner thigh muscles.
10. **Breathing**: Coordinate your breathing by inhaling during the outward swing and exhaling as you cross the leg in front of your body.
11. **Repetition**: Perform 10-15 swings on one side, switch sides, and repeat the exercise with the other leg.
12. **Mindfulness and Observation**: Throughout the leg swings, remain mindful of your body's alignment and movement. Pay attention to any areas of tightness or discomfort, and adjust the amplitude of your swings accordingly. The goal is to warm up the muscles and joints, not to push into pain.
13. **Modifications and Variations:** For an added challenge, you can perform leg swings without holding onto support, which will engage your core and improve balance. Wearing ankle weights can increase resistance and strengthen the lower body.

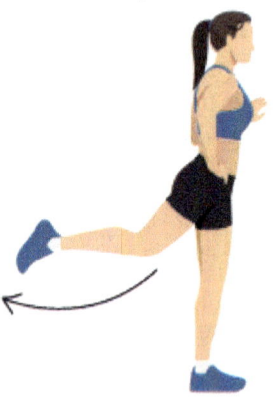

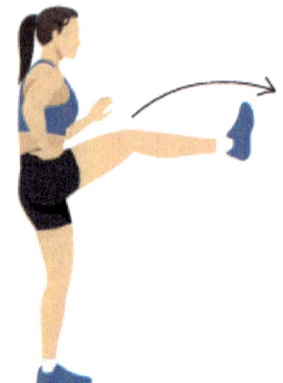

Leg swings

Gentle Squats

This foundational warm-up exercise engages and prepares the lower body, specifically the thighs, hips, and glutes, for various activities. Gentle squats focus on activating the major muscle groups involved in more downward body movement while promoting joint mobility in the knees and hips. You can effectively warm up the muscles without straining them by performing squats slowly and with a shallow depth. Here's how to perform gentle squats with attention to detail:

1. **Starting Position**: Stand with your feet shoulder-width apart or slightly wider, toes pointing slightly outward. This stance ensures stability and proper alignment during the squat. Extend your arms out in front of you for balance, or place your hands on your hips.
2. **Initiate the Squat**: Begin the movement by shifting your weight back into your heels and hinging at your hips as if you are about to sit back in a chair. Keep your chest lifted and your spine in a neutral position to prevent rounding your back.
3. **Depth and Form**: Lower your body slowly, focusing on keeping the knees aligned with your toes and not extending past them. Since this is a gentle warm-up squat, lower yourself to a shallow depth – around a quarter or half squat to avoid overloading the muscles and joints.
4. **Engage the Core**: Throughout the squat, engage your core muscles to support your lower back. This engagement is crucial for maintaining stability and ensuring the focus remains on warming the lower body.
5. **Rising**: Drive through your heels to return to the starting position, straightening your hips and knees simultaneously. Ensure the movement is smooth and controlled, using your glutes and thighs to power the ascent.
6. **Breathing**: Inhale as you lower into the squat and exhale as you rise back up. Coordinating your breath with the

movement helps maintain a rhythmic flow and encourages focus and concentration.
7. **Repetition**: Perform 10-15 gentle squats, paying attention to the quality of the movement rather than the quantity. The aim is to warm up and activate the muscles, preparing them for more strenuous activity.
8. **Mindfulness and Focus**: As you perform each squat, remain mindful of the sensations in your lower body. Notice areas of tightness or ease, using the movement to increase awareness and connection with your body.
9. **Modifications and Variations**: To modify the exercise, you can perform the squats against a wall to help maintain balance and ensure proper form. For a variation that further engages the muscles, pause at the bottom of the squat for a few seconds before rising back up.

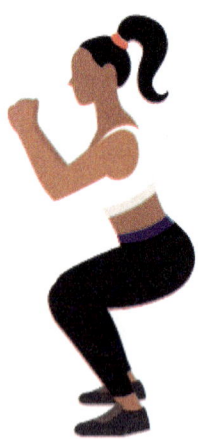

Gentle squats

Butterfly Flutters

This warm-up exercise, also known as the Butterfly Stretch, targets the inner thighs, hips, and groin area, promoting flexibility and mobility in these regions. Butterfly Flutters are particularly effective for opening up the hips and preparing the lower body for activities that require a wide range of motion. Here's a step-by-step guide to performing Butterfly Flutters correctly:

1. **Starting Position**: Begin by sitting on the floor with a straight back and engaged core. Bring the soles of your feet together in front of you, drawing them as close to your body as comfortably as possible. Grasp your feet or ankles with your hands.
2. **Knee Flutters**: Gently lower your knees towards the floor to a comfortable extent. This is your starting position. From here, lightly flutter your knees up and down, mimicking the motion of a butterfly's wings. The movement should be gentle and controlled, focusing on the sensation of opening in the hips and inner thighs.
3. **Breathing**: Coordinate your breathing with the fluttering motion, inhaling as your knees rise and exhaling as they lower. This rhythmic breathing helps facilitate muscle relaxation, allowing for a deeper stretch over time.
4. **Maintain Upright Posture**: Keep your spine long and your shoulders relaxed throughout the exercise. Resist the urge to hunch forward; instead, imagine a string pulling you up from the crown of your head, maintaining an upright and open posture.
5. **Duration and Intensity**: Continue the fluttering motion for 30 seconds to a minute, gradually slowing down towards the end of the set. The goal is to warm up and loosen the muscles and joints, not to push them to their limits.
6. **Mindfulness and Focus**: Pay attention to the sensations in your hips, inner thighs, and groin area. Notice areas of tightness or ease, and use the gentle fluttering as an opportunity to explore and release tension.
7. **Modifications and Variations**: To modify the Butterfly Stretch for more comfort or a deeper stretch, you can:
8. **Adjust the Distance**: Move your feet away from your body to lessen the intensity of the stretch or bring them closer for a deeper stretch.
9. **Add Support**: Place cushions or yoga blocks under your knees if they don't comfortably reach the floor, providing

support and allowing you to focus on relaxing into the stretch.
10. **Post-Flutter Stretch**: After completing the flutters, hold the knees down towards the ground for a static stretch, deepening the opening in the hips and inner thighs. Maintain this position for several deep breaths, allowing the muscles to relax further.

By incorporating this exercise into your warm-up routine, you can enhance your performance in activities that demand flexibility and strength in the hips and legs.

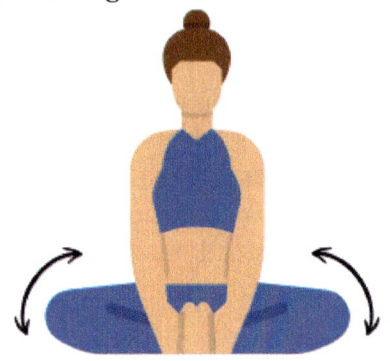

Butterfly Flutters

Standing Calf Raises

This targeted warm-up exercise activates and prepares the calf muscles (gastrocnemius and soleus) for various activities, enhancing their strength, flexibility, and endurance. By lifting and lowering the heels, you warm up the calves and promote ankle stability and mobility. Here's a detailed guide to performing standing Calf raises effectively:
1. **Starting Position**: Stand with your feet hip-width apart, ensuring your toes point forward and your weight is evenly distributed. You can perform this exercise near a wall or a sturdy piece of furniture to lightly hold onto for balance if needed.

2. **Engage Your Core**: Before initiating the movement, engage your core muscles to stabilize your torso and prevent unnecessary swaying or leaning forward. Keep your shoulders relaxed and down.
3. **Lift Your Heels**: Begin the exercise by slowly lifting your heels off the ground and pressing up onto the balls of your feet. Focus on using the strength of your calf muscles to execute the lift rather than bouncing or using momentum. Aim to reach the highest point of elevation that feels comfortable, ensuring you maintain balance and control.
4. **Pause and Stretch**: Once you've lifted your heels as high as possible, pause at the top of the movement for a second. You should feel a stretch through your calves and a contraction in the muscles as they work to hold your body up.
5. **Lower with Control**: Slowly lower your heels to the ground, maintaining control throughout the descent. The lowering phase is as important as the lifting, as it helps lengthen the calf muscles and improve flexibility.
6. **Breathing**: Coordinate your breath with the movement by inhaling as you lower your heels and exhaling as you lift. Proper breathing helps maintain a rhythmic pattern and ensures adequate oxygen flow to the working muscles.
7. **Repetition**: Perform 10-15 calf raises, focusing on the quality of the movement rather than speed. As your calves warm up, you can lift your heels or feel more stretch and muscle engagement.
8. **Mindfulness and Focus**: Pay close attention to how your calves feel during the exercise. Notice areas of tightness, strength, or flexibility, using the exercise to increase awareness and connection with your lower body.
9. **Modifications and Variations**: To increase the challenge or vary the stimulus to the calves, you can:

    - **Single-Leg Calf Raises**: Perform the exercise on one leg at a time, adding a balance component and intensifying each Calf's work.

- **Elevated Calf Raises**: Stand with the balls of your feet on a raised surface (like a step or a curb) with your heels hanging off the edge. This variation increases the range of motion, providing a deeper stretch and more muscular contraction.

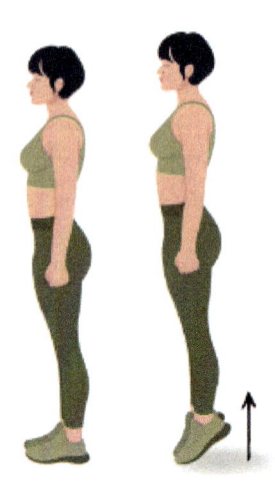

Standing Calf Raises

3.2 Core Somatic Movements

This section is the heart of your journey, where the essence of somatic exercises unfolds through movements designed to enhance body awareness, release chronic tension, and cultivate a harmonious balance between the mind, body, and spirit.

Core somatic movements are about connecting deeply with yourself, exploring the subtleties of your body's language, and using gentle, mindful movements to foster physical and emotional well-being. These exercises are not just physical acts but a form of communication with the inner self, encouraging introspection, healing, and growth.

Introduction to Core Somatic Movements

Each movement in this section is a key to unlocking areas of stiffness, discomfort, or disconnection, allowing you to regain control, flexibility, and strength. You'll be guided step-by-step through each exercise, learning to perform them with intention and sensitivity to your body's unique needs and responses.

Let's start!

Pelvic Clocks

This exercise is a fundamental somatic movement designed to increase your awareness and control of the pelvic area, affecting your entire spine's alignment and mobility. By envisioning your pelvis as a clock face, you can explore subtle pelvic tilts and shifts that engage different muscles and connective tissues, promoting flexibility, stability, and ease of movement. Here's how to perform Pelvic Clocks with precision:

Understanding the Pelvic Clock:

Visualize the Clock: Imagine the pelvis as a clock face lying horizontally. The navel or belly button represents 12 o'clock, the pubic bone is 6 o'clock, and the two hip bones are 3 and 9 o'clock, respectively.

Starting Position:
- **Initial Setup**: Lie on a comfortable surface with your knees bent and feet flat on the floor, hip-width apart. Place your arms by your sides with palms facing down. This neutral position allows for optimal movement of the pelvis.

Performing the Exercise:
1. **12 to 6 Movement**: Gently tilt your pelvis towards your head, moving the navel upwards to 12 o'clock, which flattens the lower back against the floor. Then, list the pelvis towards your feet, moving the pubic bone to 6 o'clock and slightly arching your lower back. This anterior and posterior pelvic tilt warms the spine and engages the core.
2. **3 to 9 Movement**: Shift your weight to one hip, rolling it towards 3 o'clock, then gently shift to the opposite hip,

moving towards 9 o'clock. This lateral tilting action activates the oblique muscles and mobilizes the hips and lower back.
3. **Circular Motion**: Combine the movements by circling the pelvis in a smooth, continuous motion around the clock face. Start in one direction, gently hitting each " hour, " then reverse the direction, ensuring balanced engagement and mobility.
4. **Breathing**: Coordinate your breath with the movement, inhaling as you move to one extreme of the clock and exhaling as you pass through another. This synchronization enhances the effectiveness of the exercise and promotes relaxation.
5. **Mindfulness and Sensation**: Pay close attention to your pelvic region and lower back sensations. Notice areas of tension, ease, or particular sensitivity. The goal is to cultivate a deeper awareness of your pelvic movements and their impact on your posture and spinal health.
6. **Frequency and Duration**: Perform the Pelvic Clocks for 1-2 minutes, exploring each direction and combination of movements. Focus on the quality of movement rather than speed, allowing your awareness and control to deepen with each rotation.

Benefits:
- **Enhanced Pelvic Mobility**: Regular practice of Pelvic Clocks can lead to increased mobility and flexibility in the pelvic area and lower back, contributing to improved posture and movement efficiency.
- **Spinal Health**: By promoting subtle adjustments and alignments within the pelvic region, you can positively affect the health of your entire spine, potentially alleviating discomfort and stiffness in the back.
- **Core Engagement**: This exercise naturally engages and strengthens the core muscles, including the deep stabilizers of the spine, which are crucial for overall stability and strength.

- This exercise promotes nuanced control and awareness of the pelvic region.

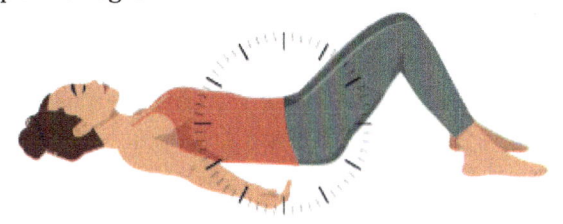

Pelvic clock

Arch and Flatten

This exercise is a cornerstone in somatic practices for its simplicity and profound impact on spinal health. It teaches you to gently articulate your spine, moving between flexion and extension, which can help release tension in the back muscles, improve spinal fluidity, and enhance overall posture. Here's a detailed guide to performing the Arch and Flatten exercise effectively:

Starting Position:
- **Initial Setup**: Lie on your back on a comfortable surface, such as a yoga mat, with your knees bent and feet flat on the floor, hip-width apart. Let your arms rest by your sides with palms facing down. This position allows your spine to be in a neutral alignment, ready for movement.

Performing the Exercise:
1. **Flatten Phase**: Begin by exhaling and engaging your abdominal muscles to press the small of your back into the floor. This action flattens the spine against the ground, creating a gentle posterior pelvic tilt. As you flatten your back, focus on the sensation of the floor pressing against your spine, encouraging the release of tension in the lower back muscles.
2. **Arch Phase**: Inhale and slowly release the engagement of your abdominal muscles, allowing your lower back to arch off the floor. This introduces an anterior pelvic tilt,

creating space between your lower back and the floor. The movement should be controlled and gentle, focusing on the natural curvature of the lumbar spine.
3. **Coordination with Breath**: The Arch and Flatten exercise closely coordinates with your breathing pattern. Exhale as you flatten your back, pressing the spine into the floor, and inhale as you arch your back, creating space. This breathwork enhances the movement's effectiveness, promoting relaxation and deeper muscle engagement.
4. **Mindfulness and Sensation**: Remember the sensations in your spine and surrounding muscles throughout the exercise. Notice areas of tightness, mobility, or ease as you move through the arching and flattening phases. The goal is to cultivate a deeper awareness of your spinal movements and to encourage a dialogue between your body and your breath.
5. **Repetition and Rhythm**: Continue to alternate between arching and flattening your back for several cycles, typically for 1-2 minutes. Establish a smooth rhythm that mirrors the natural flow of your breath, allowing each movement to transition into the next seamlessly.
6. **Modifications and Variations**: For individuals with significant back discomfort or those seeking a more profound engagement, placing a small, rolled-up towel under the lower back during the flattening phase can provide additional support and feedback for the movement.

Benefits:
- **Engages the Entire Core Musculature**: The movement between spinal flexion (arching) and extension (flattening) engages the superficial muscles and the deeper core muscles surrounding the spine. This includes the rectus abdominis, the obliques, the transverse abdominis, and the multifidus. Engaging these muscles helps to strengthen the core, providing better stability and support for the entire body.

- **Spinal Mobility**: Regularly performing the Arch and Flatten exercise can significantly improve your spine's mobility, encouraging flexibility and reducing the risk of stiffness and discomfort.
- **Muscle Relaxation**: This exercise effectively releases tension in the back muscles, particularly in the lumbar region, which is often tight due to prolonged sitting or standing.
- **Postural Awareness**: By engaging in the gentle articulation of the spine, you become more aware of your posture during exercise and daily life. This awareness can improve how you carry yourself, potentially alleviating postural-related discomfort.

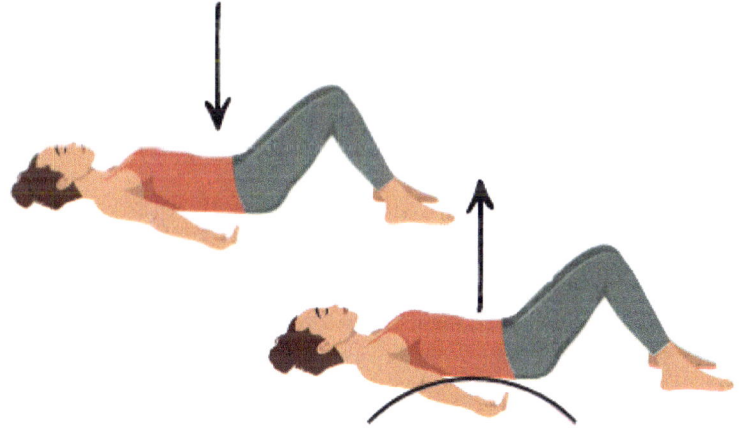

Arch and Flatten

Hamstring Lengthening

Tight hamstrings are common for many people, often contributing to lower back discomfort and limiting mobility. The Hamstring Lengthening exercise in somatic practices focuses on gently releasing this tightness, enhancing flexibility, and promoting a sense of ease and fluidity in the legs. Unlike traditional static stretching, this approach encourages a mindful and gradual increase in length and flexibility of the hamstrings, minimizing strain. Here's how to perform the Hamstring Lengthening exercise with attention to detail.

Preparation:
- **Initial Setup**: Find a comfortable space on your back, preferably on a yoga mat or a soft, flat surface. Keep a yoga strap, belt, or towel within reach.

Performing the Exercise:
1. **Starting Position**: Lie on your back with both legs extended and arms resting by your sides. Begin with a few deep breaths to center yourself and prepare your body for the exercise.
2. **Bend One Knee**: Gently bend your right knee, bringing the foot flat on the floor. This position stabilizes your pelvis and protects your lower back during the stretch.
3. **Introduce the Strap**: Place the yoga strap, belt, or towel around the arch of your left foot (the leg is still extended on the floor). Hold the ends of the strap in both hands. This tool will help you gently guide the movement without straining.
4. **Lift and Lengthen**: Gradually straighten your left leg towards the ceiling, holding the strap securely. Keep a slight bend in the knee to avoid hyperextension. Adjust the tension on the belt to find a comfortable stretch in your hamstring. The goal is not to forcefully pull the leg towards you but to allow the weight of the portion and the gentle guidance of the strap to lengthen the muscle.
5. **Mindful Movement**: Focus on breathing deeply as you hold the position, encouraging the hamstring to relax and lengthen with each exhale. Rather than aiming for maximum flexibility, the aim is to explore the sensation of lengthening and releasing tension in the muscle.
6. **Adjustment and Observation**: If you feel a significant stretch, maintain the position, breathing into the sensation. If the sensation diminishes, you can gently increase the stretch by pulling lightly on the strap or extending the leg more towards you. Maintain a mindful approach, always listening to your body's feedback.

7. **Duration**: Hold the stretch for 30 seconds to a minute, then slowly release the leg back to the starting position. Take a moment to observe any differences in sensation between the two legs.
8. **Switch Sides**: Repeat the process with your right leg, ensuring both sides receive equal attention to promote balance and symmetry in flexibility.

Benefits:
- **Pelvic Stability and Alignment**: The hamstrings attach from the ischial tuberosity of the pelvis down to the lower leg. When they are tight, they can pull the pelvis into a posterior tilt (backward rotation), flattening the lower back and disrupting the spine's natural alignment. Lengthening the hamstrings reduces this rear pull on the pelvis, promoting a more neutral pelvic position. A neutral pelvis supports the optimal engagement and functioning of the core muscles, enhancing stability and posture.
- **Reduced Back Discomfort**: By addressing tightness in the hamstrings, this exercise can also help alleviate tension in the lower back, often a side effect of tight hamstrings.
- **Enhanced Body Awareness**: This gentle approach to stretching encourages a deeper connection with your body, fostering an understanding of how mindful movement can influence physical sensations and well-being.
- Hamstring Lengthening is a foundational exercise in somatic practices, embodying the principles of awareness, gentle movement, and the body's natural capacity for change and improvement. Through consistent practice, you can achieve greater flexibility and a deeper sense of ease in your legs, contributing to overall physical and emotional balance.

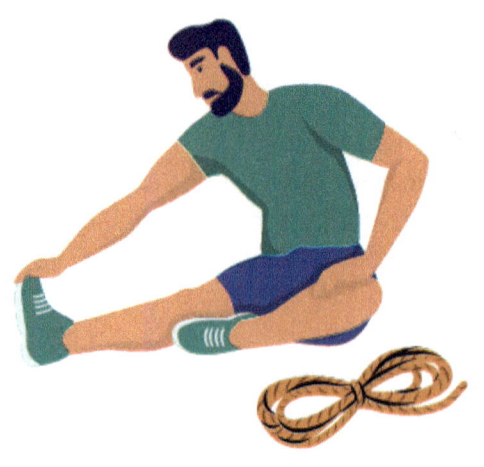

Hamstring Lengthening

<u>Side Bends</u>

Side Bends are a fundamental exercise in enhancing lateral (side-to-side) flexibility in the spine and ribcage, which is crucial for overall spinal health and mobility and enhances breath capacity. This exercise targets the lateral core muscles, including the obliques, intercostals (muscles between the ribs), and quadratus lumborum, contributing significantly to the core's strength and flexibility. Here's a detailed guide to performing Side Bends effectively and understanding their importance for core improvement:

Performing Side Bends:
1. **Starting Position**: Stand with your feet hip-width apart, ensuring stable grounding. Keep your knees slightly bent to avoid locking them, maintaining a natural, supportive base.
2. **Initiate the Bend**: Extend your arms overhead by clasping your hands together or holding them parallel. Keeping your hips and shoulders facing forward, inhale deeply.
3. **Bend to the Side**: As you exhale, gently bend your torso to one side (say, to the right), pushing your left hip out slightly. The movement should originate from the waist,

focusing on creating length along the side of your body rather than merely leaning over it. Keep both feet firmly planted to avoid tilting.
4. **Deepening the Stretch**: Reach actively through your fingertips to intensify the stretch along your entire side, from the hip through the ribcage and up to the arms. Ensure your head is in a neutral position, aligned with your spine.
5. **Return to Center**: Inhale and slowly return to the starting position, feeling the elongation in your spine.
6. **Repeat on the Opposite Side**: Perform the side bend on the other side to maintain balance in flexibility and strength across your body.
7. **Why It's Important for Core Improvement?**
8. Side Bends directly engage and strengthen the lateral core muscles, particularly the obliques. Strong obliques are essential for rotational movements, lateral stability, and spine protection during daily activities and athletic endeavors.

Add weight when the exercise becomes too light.

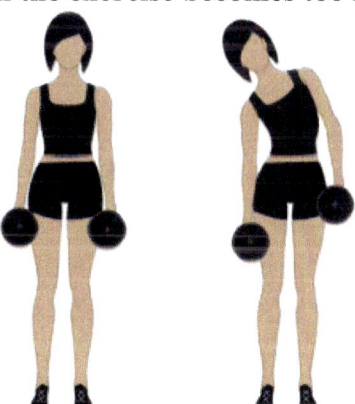

Side bends

Cat Stretch Sequence

This dynamic exercise is an expansion of the traditional cat-cow stretch, incorporating additional movements to explore spinal flexion, extension, and rotation deeply. It serves as a comprehensive spinal warm-up, engaging the muscles along the spine and enhancing core strength and flexibility. Here's a step-by-step guide to performing the Cat Stretch Sequence with attention to detail:

The Position:
1. **Initial Setup**: Begin on a comfortable, flat surface on your hands and knees. Position your knees directly under your hips and your wrists under your shoulders. Spread your fingers wide for stability, and start with a neutral spine.
2. **Cow Pose (Spinal Extension)**: Inhale as you drop your belly towards the floor, lifting your sit bones and chest toward the ceiling, and gently raise your head to look forward or slightly up. This position encourages spinal extension.
3. **Cat Pose (Spinal Flexion)**: Exhale as you draw your belly to your spine, rounding your back toward the ceiling and tucking your chin to your chest. This position emphasizes spinal flexion.
4. Additional Movements:
5. **Side-to-Side Flexion**: Return to a neutral spine. Begin gently shifting your hips to one side, then to the other, creating a lateral bending in the spine. This movement adds a side-to-side flexion component, warming the lateral muscles and increasing spinal mobility.
6. **Circular Movements**: Introduce circular movements to *the spine by combining the cat-cow stretch with the side*-to-side flexion. Move your spine in a circular motion, arching up into cat pose as you round the back, then dipping down into cow pose as you lower the belly. Incorporate the lateral flexion by weaving in the side shifts. Perform the circles in one direction, then reverse. This enhances the range of motion and engages the core muscles dynamically.
7. **Thread the Needle (Spinal Rotation)**: From the neutral position, slide your right arm underneath your left, lowering your right shoulder and cheek to the floor. This

adds a rotational component to the sequence, stretching the shoulders and further mobilizing the thoracic spine. Hold a few breaths, then unwind and repeat on the other side.

Benefits:
- **Core Engagement**: The Cat Stretch Sequence actively engages the core muscles throughout the various movements, strengthening the abdominals, obliques, and lower back muscles. This engagement is crucial for spinal stability and overall core strength.
- **Postural Benefits**: Regular practice of this sequence can improve posture by balancing muscular strength and flexibility around the spine and core, reducing the risk of back pain and muscular imbalances.

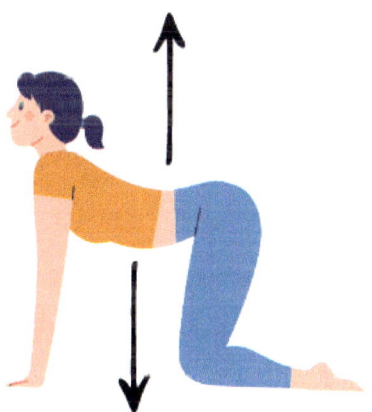

Cat Stretch Sequence

Constructive Rest Position

This is a foundational somatic posture revered for promoting deep relaxation and awareness and serving as a gateway for more profound somatic explorations. This position is particularly beneficial for the core for several reasons, focusing on reducing tension, aligning the spine, and facilitating a natural balance within the body's central structure.

How to Perform Constructive Rest Position:
1. **Finding the Position**: Lie on your back on a comfortable, flat surface. Bend your knees and place your feet flat, hip-width apart. Let your arms rest by your sides, palms facing up or down based on comfort.
2. **Aligning the Spine**: Ensure your spine is in a neutral position, with its natural curves present but not exaggerated. The goal is to allow the floor to support your body fully, minimizing the effort to hold any particular posture.
3. **Settling In**: Close your eyes and take a few deep breaths, allowing your body to relax deeply into the floor with each exhale. Focus on releasing unnecessary tension, particularly in the back, hips, and shoulders.
4. **Duration**: Stay in this position for 5-10 minutes, using the time to cultivate an awareness of your body's sensations and the subtle movements of your breath.

Benefits:
- **Stress and Tension Release**: The Constructive Rest Position allows the core muscles, including the deeper stabilizing muscles, to relax and release stored tension. This relaxation is crucial for restoring balance and function to the core muscles, which are often overtaxed by daily activities and poor posture.
- **Spinal Alignment**: By supporting the spine's natural curvature against a flat surface, this position encourages the alignment of the spinal column. Proper alignment reduces strain on the core muscles and facilitates a more efficient and balanced engagement.
- **Pelvic Floor Activation**: The bent knees and relaxed posture help subtly activate the pelvic floor muscles, which are integral to core stability and strength. This gentle activation fosters awareness and control of these often-neglected muscles.
- **Foundation for Movement Exploration**: Any subsequent movement or exercise is performed from a more centered

and balanced foundation by starting in a state of relaxation and alignment. This ensures that core engagement and spinal alignment are optimized in more dynamic somatic practices.

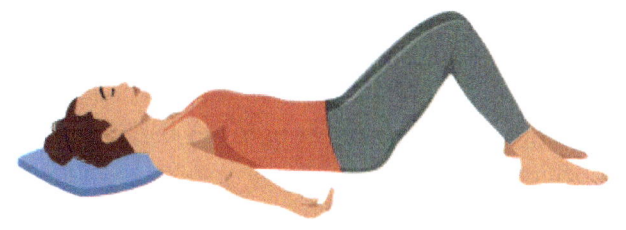

Constructive Rest Position

Hip Joint Release

Hip Joint involves a series of gentle, mindful movements designed to increase flexibility, reduce tension, and improve the range of motion in the hip joints. This exercise benefits the hips and the core, as the two are intrinsically linked in supporting the body's movement and stability. Here's a detailed guide to performing the Hip Joint Release and its significance for core strength and health.

How to Perform Hip Joint Release:
1. **Starting Position**: Lie on your back on a comfortable surface with extended legs. Relax your arms by your sides, palms facing down, to maintain a neutral spine.
2. **Knee-to-Chest**: Gently bend one knee and bring it towards your chest, clasping your hands around your shin or the back of your thigh. Keep the other leg straight and grounded. This initial movement starts the process of opening the hip on one side.
3. **Circling the Leg**: Holding the knee, make small circles with the hip joint. Start with small circles, gradually increasing the radius as your hip loosens. This circling motion helps to lubricate the hip joint, promoting greater mobility.

4. **Switch Directions**: After several circles in one direction, pause and then switch, circling the knee in the opposite direction to ensure even hip joint mobilization.
5. **Leg Extension and Flexion**: Extend the leg upward, holding it with both hands behind the thigh or calf (avoid putting pressure on the knee). Gently flex and extend the foot to stretch the hamstring and calf muscles, further promoting hip mobility through the connectedness of the leg muscles.
6. **Repeat on the Other Side**: After completing the sequence on one side, gently lower the leg back to the starting position and repeat the exercise with the other leg to ensure balanced hip mobility.

Benefits:
- **Pelvic Stability**: The hips are directly connected to the pelvic region, the foundation for core stability. By releasing tension and increasing mobility in the hips, the pelvic muscles can function more efficiently, enhancing the overall stability and strength of the core.
- **Improved Posture**: These exercises help correct these imbalances by allowing the hips to move freely, supporting a more upright and balanced posture.
- **Breathing and Core Activation**: Focusing on gentle, controlled movements encourages deep, diaphragmatic breathing, which inherently engages and strengthens the core muscles, particularly the deep stabilizers of the spine.
-

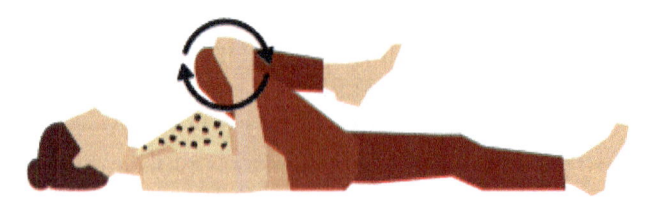

Hip joint release

Twisting from the Core

This exercise promotes gentle spinal rotation, essential for improving spinal flexibility, enhancing core strength, and correcting asymmetries in the body. Spinal twists engage and challenge the core muscles, including the obliques, rectus abdominis, and deep stabilizers of the spine, making them an integral component of a comprehensive core conditioning program. Here's a detailed guide to performing Twisting from the core effectively and understanding its benefits:

How to Perform Twisting from the Core:
1. **Starting Position**: Sit on the floor with your legs extended or cross-legged, depending on your flexibility and comfort. Ensure your spine is erect and your shoulders relaxed away from your ears.
2. **Initiate the Twist**: Bend your right knee and place your right foot outside your left knee. If sitting with legs extended, you can keep the left leg straight or bend it so your left foot tucks near your right buttock for a more profound twist.
3. **Engage the Twist**: Place your right hand on the floor behind you for support. Inhale to lengthen your spine, and twist your torso to the right as you exhale. Bring your left elbow to the outside of your right knee as a lever to deepen the twist, ensuring the movement originates from the core.
4. **Breathing and Deepening**: With each inhalation, focus on lengthening the spine further; gently deepen the twist with each exhalation. This rhythmic breathing helps maximize the stretch and engagement of the core muscles.
5. **Hold and Focus**: Maintain the twist for 20-30 seconds, concentrating on your core and spine sensations. Avoid forcing the twist; instead, allow the depth of the wrench to increase naturally with each breath.
6. **Release and Repeat**: Gently unwind the twist, returning to your starting position. Repeat the twist on the opposite side to ensure balanced engagement and flexibility in the core and spine.

Benefits:

- **Oblique Strengthening**: Twisting movements directly engage and strengthen the oblique muscles, which are crucial for rotational movements, lateral stability, and protecting the spine during daily activities and athletic endeavors.
- **Corrects Asymmetries**: Regular practice of spinal twists can help address and correct asymmetries in the body by evenly stretching and strengthening the core muscles on both sides of the body. This balance is essential for proper posture and alignment.
- **Enhances Digestion and Detoxification**: The twisting motion massages the internal organs, stimulating digestion and detoxification processes. A healthy digestive system supports core strength and health by reducing bloating and abdominal discomfort.

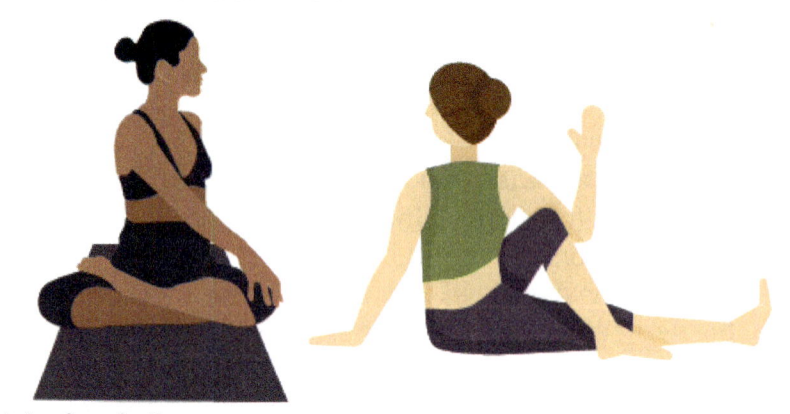

Twisting from the Core

Diaphragmatic Breathing Exploration

This exercise involves deep, focused breathing that engages the diaphragm, a large muscle at the base of the lungs. Diaphragmatic breathing is crucial for effective respiratory function and is significant in core stability and strength. Practicing diaphragmatic breathing can improve oxygen exchange, reduce stress levels, and enhance core muscle function. Here's a detailed guide to performing Diaphragmatic Breathing Exploration and understanding its benefits for the core:

How to Perform Diaphragmatic Breathing Exploration:
1. **Find a Comfortable Position**: Begin by lying on your back, sitting comfortably, or standing with good posture. The key is to be in a position where your chest and abdomen are not restricted.
2. **Place Your Hands for Feedback**: Put one hand on your upper chest and the other on your belly. This placement will help you feel the movement of your diaphragm and ensure that you are breathing correctly.
3. **Inhale Through the Nose**: Slowly inhale through your nose, focusing on directing the breath downwards so that your belly rises under your hand. The hand on your chest should remain relatively still, indicating that the movement is coming from your diaphragm rather than your chest muscles.
4. **Exhale Through the Mouth**: Gently exhale through your mouth, feeling the belly fall. As you exhale, engage your core muscles slightly, as if gently hugging your spine with your belly. This engagement enhances the exercise's benefit to the core.
5. **Focus on the Breath**: Continue to breathe deeply and slowly, concentrating on the rise and fall of your belly. Aim for smooth, even breaths, gradually lengthening both the inhalation and exhalation as you become more comfortable with the technique.
6. **Practice Regularly**: Diaphragmatic breathing can be practiced multiple times throughout the day. Regular practice is key to retraining your breathing pattern and strengthening your diaphragm and core muscles.

Benefits:
- **Core Muscle Engagement**: The diaphragm is intrinsically linked to the core muscles, including the transverse abdominis, pelvic floor, multifidus, and obliques. Activating the diaphragm through deep breathing stimulates these muscles, contributing to a stronger, more stable core.

- **Enhances Oxygenation and Performance**: By improving the efficiency of your breathing, diaphragmatic breathing exploration increases oxygenation to your muscles, including the core muscles. Better oxygenation can enhance endurance and performance in physical activities.
- **Reduces Stress and Tension**: Deep, controlled breathing calms the nervous system, reducing stress and tension that can accumulate in the core muscles. A relaxed core is more flexible and functions more effectively.
- **Facilitates Mind-Body Connection**: This breathing practice fosters increased awareness of the body's internal state, enhancing the mind-body connection. A heightened awareness of the core region can improve the effectiveness of other core exercises and daily movements.

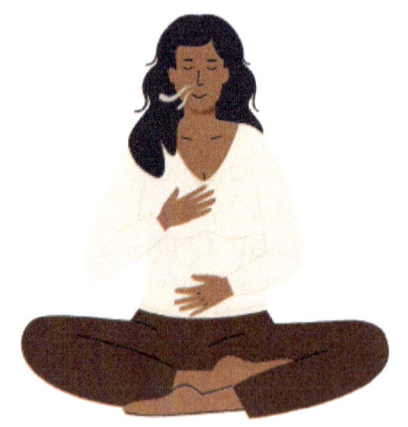

Diaphragmatic Breathing Exploration

<u>Rolling Bridge</u>

The Rolling Bridge is an exercise that combines the principles of movement fluidity with core and spinal stabilization. It involves a sequential lifting of the spine off the ground, segment by segment, into a bridge position, followed by a controlled rolling back down to the starting position. This exercise mobilizes the spine and strengthens the core, glutes, and hamstrings. Here's a detailed guide to performing the Rolling Bridge and its benefits for the core:

Performing the Rolling Bridge:
1. **Starting Position**: Lie on your back on a comfortable surface with your knees bent and feet flat on the floor, hip-width apart. Place your arms by your sides with palms facing down for support.
2. **Initiate the Lift**: Begin by gently engaging your core muscles to tilt your pelvis, flattening the lower back against the floor. This initial pelvic tilt is crucial for activating the deep core muscles and protecting the spine as you move into the bridge.
3. **Sequential Lifting**: Continue to lift your hips off the floor by pressing down through your feet, starting with the tailbone and moving up the spine, one vertebra at a time, until your body forms a straight line from your shoulders to your knees. Focus on peeling each spine segment off the floor in a smooth, rolling motion.
4. **Peak of the Bridge**: Once in the full bridge position, ensure that your glutes and hamstrings are engaged and your core is stable. Avoid overarching the lower back by maintaining a firm engagement of the abdominal muscles.
5. **Rolling Down**: Begin the descent by reversing the lifting sequence, starting from the upper spine and moving down, vertebra by vertebra, until the tailbone gently touches the floor last. This controlled rolling motion emphasizes spinal articulation and core engagement.
6. **Breathing**: Inhale as you prepare to lift into the bridge, and exhale as you roll your spine back down to the floor. Proper breathing enhances core activation and supports the smooth execution of the exercise.
7. **Repetitions**: Perform 8-12 repetitions of the Rolling Bridge, focusing on the quality of movement and maintaining core engagement throughout the exercise.

Benefits:

- **Deep Core Activation**: The Rolling Bridge exercise requires a continuous engagement of the deep core muscles, including the transverse abdominis and pelvic floor, throughout the lifting and lowering phases. This engagement strengthens the core and improves stability.
- **Spinal Articulation**: The segmental movement of the spine during the exercise enhances spinal health and flexibility. A flexible spine supported by a strong core contributes to improved posture and reduces the risk of back pain.
- **Balance and Coordination**: Maintaining stability during the bridge position challenges the core's ability to stabilize the body against gravity. This balance and coordination work strengthens the core and improves overall body control.
- **Synergistic Muscle Engagement**: The exercise involves the glutes and hamstrings, which are key to supporting the lower back and core. Strengthening these muscles with the core creates a more integrated and functional support system for the spine and pelvis.
- **Stress Reduction**: The focused, mindful movement of the Rolling Bridge, combined with synchronized breathing, can have a calming effect, reducing physical and mental stress. A relaxed body is more conducive to effective core engagement and overall well-being.

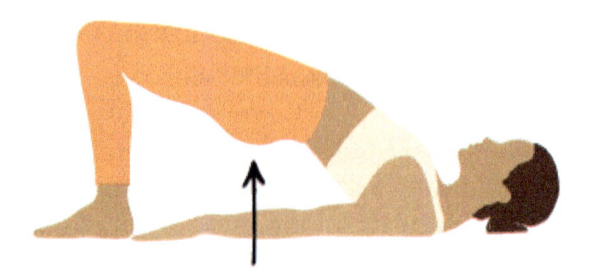

Rolling Bridge

Chapter 4: Mindful Practices for Emotional Balance

In this Chapter, we embark on a transformative journey towards achieving serenity and stability through "Mindfulness and Meditation." This section delves into the heart of mindfulness and meditation practices, indispensable tools for cultivating emotional balance and mitigating stress. The essence of mindfulness lies in maintaining a moment-by-moment awareness of our thoughts, feelings, bodily sensations, and the surrounding environment with an attitude of openness, curiosity, and acceptance.

4.1 Mindfulness and Meditation:

Mindfulness meditation begins with the breath, the life force that moves within us yet often goes unnoticed. By directing your focus to your breathing, you can anchor yourself in the present moment, a fundamental step in reducing the cacophony of stress and the whirlwind of daily thoughts. The practice does not require a specific belief system or spiritual alignment; it is a universal tool for improving mental clarity, emotional stability, and physical well-being.

Techniques to Cultivate Mindfulness and Meditation:
- **Focused Breathing:** Find a quiet, comfortable place to sit or lie down. Close your eyes and bring your attention to your breath, noticing the sensation of air entering and leaving your nostrils or the rise and fall of your chest. When your mind wanders, gently bring your focus back to your breath. This practice helps center your thoughts and calms the mind.
- **Body Scan Meditation:** This technique involves mentally scanning your body for areas of tension and consciously relaxing these areas. Beginning at your feet and moving upwards, pay attention to each part of your body. This promotes bodily awareness and enhances the connection

between mind and body, which is crucial for emotional balance.
- **Mindful Observation:** Choose an object from nature and focus on observing it for a few minutes. This could be a flower, an insect, or the moon. Notice every detail about it: its color, shape, and texture. This practice of focused observation encourages a connection with the present moment and the larger world.
- **Mindful Listening:** Listen to the sounds in your environment or a piece of music, paying attention to every note or nuance. This helps develop an acute awareness of the present and fosters a deep engagement with your surroundings, reducing stress and enhancing focus.

Connecting Mindfulness to Physical Movement
As we transition to "4.2 Connecting Exercise to Mindfulness," it becomes evident that mindfulness and physical activity are intrinsically linked. The principles of mindfulness applied to exercise transform physical activities into meditative practices. By focusing on the body's movement and the sensation of each breath during exercise, you can deepen your mindfulness practice, creating a holistic approach to well-being that nourishes both the body and mind. This symbiotic relationship between movement and mindfulness paves the way for a deeper exploration of how somatic exercises and mindful practices can be integrated to promote a harmonious balance between physical and emotional well-being.

Through "Mindfulness and Meditation," you are equipped with the foundational tools to navigate the complexities of emotions and stress, setting the stage for a comprehensive exploration of mindfulness in movement and daily life. This journey enhances emotional balance and enriches your overall quality of life, embodying the essence of harmonizing the physical and emotional self.

4.2 Mindfulness and Meditation:

Integrating mindfulness into somatic exercises transforms physical movements into a powerful conduit for more profound emotional release and awareness. Now we start exploring the seamless fusion of mindful practices with physical activities, creating a holistic approach that amplifies both benefits. This integration enhances physical flexibility and strength and promotes a profound sense of mental clarity and emotional balance.

The essence of mindfulness — being fully present and engaged at the moment, with a non-judgmental awareness of our thoughts, feelings, and bodily sensations — aligns perfectly with the principles of somatic exercises. These exercises, which focus on the internal movement experience, provide an ideal framework for practicing mindfulness.

1. **Start with Intention**: Before beginning your somatic exercise routine, take a moment to set an intention for your practice. This could be focusing on releasing tension in a specific body area, cultivating a sense of calm, or simply being present. This intention-setting helps to direct your focus and deepen the connection between mind and body.
2. **Breath as the Anchor**: Utilize your breath as the central focus throughout your exercise. Please pay attention to the rhythm of your breathing, how it changes with different movements, and how it feels in other parts of your body. Breathing consciously and with awareness enhances the mindfulness aspect of your practice and supports deeper emotional release.
3. **Engage Fully with Each Movement**: As you perform each somatic exercise, bring your full attention to the sensations in your body. Notice the stretch in your muscles, the alignment of your bones, and any areas of tension or ease. By fully engaging with each movement, you cultivate a heightened sense of bodily awareness, a cornerstone of mindfulness.

4. **Observe Without Judgment**: Mindfulness encourages observation without judgment. As you notice sensations, thoughts, or emotions arising during your practice, acknowledge them without criticism. This acceptance attitude helps foster emotional release and healing, allowing you to process and let go of stored emotions.
5. **Conclude with Reflection**: After completing your somatic exercise session, take a few moments to reflect on your experience. Observe any changes in your physical or emotional state, acknowledging the work you've done. This reflection period is integral to integrating mindfulness into your practice, allowing for a deeper understanding of the interplay between physical movement and emotional well-being.

Integrating mindfulness into somatic exercises sets the stage for deeper **self-exploration**. Journaling about your experiences during mindful bodily activities can provide invaluable insights into your emotional landscape, helping to identify patterns, triggers, and pathways to healing. This written reflection complements the physical practice, offering a comprehensive emotional balance and well-being approach.

Integrating mindfulness into somatic exercises allows you to embark on a transformative journey that transcends physical benefits, touching the depths of emotional release and awareness.

4.3 Journaling for Emotional Awareness:

Delves into the transformative practice of journaling as a tool to enhance self-awareness and emotional intelligence. Keeping a journal documenting progress, emotions, and bodily sensations creates a tangible record of your journey toward emotional balance and physical well-being. This practice encourages a reflective and introspective approach to personal growth, allowing you to identify patterns, celebrate achievements, and navigate challenges with greater insight.

Creating Your Journal for Emotional and Physical Tracking

Start with a Simple Notebook: Choose a notebook that resonates with you. It can be as straightforward or as elaborate as you like. The key is that it invites you to write.

Daily Entries: Dedicate a few minutes daily to jot down your experiences. You can start by noting any somatic exercises you practiced, the emotions you felt before and after the session, and any specific bodily sensations that arose during the practice.

Reflect on Progress: Regularly, at the end of each week, reflect on your entries. Note any changes or patterns in your emotional state, physical sensations, and overall well-being.

Download your Tracking Journal for your exercises.

To further enrich your experience and provide a structured way to keep track of your progress, as a gift with this book is a complete journal that can be downloaded via **QR code:**

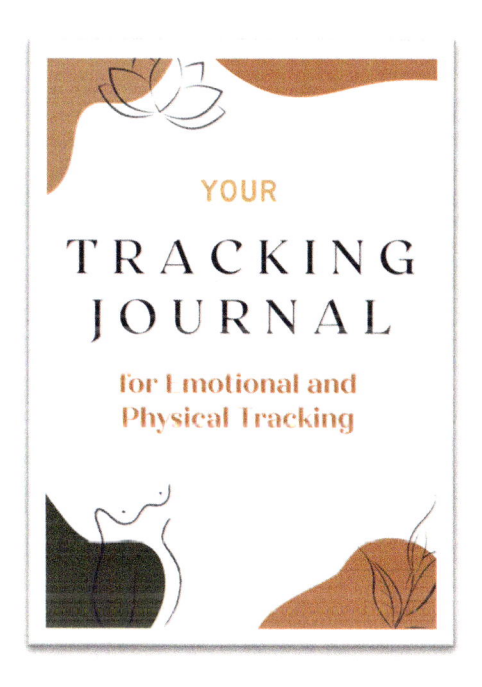

This carefully designed Journal will be your companion to ensure that the exercises shared in this book fit seamlessly into your daily life.

We recommend printing it out to fill it out more efficiently and carrying it conveniently.

The Journal is a structured 4-week program that includes all exercises and your feedback, day by day. It's a tracker and a reflection tool to jot down comments before and after each workout. This reflection process is invaluable to observing your growth, understanding your body's responses, and making necessary changes for a personalized practice.

The journey continues beyond these pages. If this book and the Tracking Journal have enriched your path to wellness, share your experience with a **review on Amazon**. Leave your review on Amazon and light the way for other seekers of health and harmony.

Thanks in advance ☺

Chapter 5: Nutritional Insights for Weight Loss

5.1 Basic Nutrition Principles:

In Chapter 5, we transition seamlessly from mindful movement and emotional balance to the foundational aspect of physical well-being: nutrition. "5.1 Basic Nutrition Principles" serves as your gateway to understanding the critical role of a balanced diet in supporting weight loss, enhancing health, and complementing your somatic practice.

Without a doubt, maintaining a well-balanced diet is essential for achieving and maintaining optimal health. Consuming various foods in the appropriate proportions is crucial to achieving and sustaining a healthy body weight and supporting overall well-being. A balanced diet is essential for proper bodily function, physical recovery, and energy maintenance. Empower yourself to take control of your health with a balanced diet. With each nutrient-dense meal, we nourish our bodies, fuel our minds, and inspire ourselves to live our best lives. So, let's strive for balance in our diets and embrace the endless possibilities of a healthier, happier life. In this context, we delve into the fundamental components of a balanced diet and why it is crucial for weight loss and overall health. Here, we explore the key elements of a balanced diet and why it's indispensable for weight loss and health.

Macronutrients: The Big Three

1. **Carbohydrates**: Often misunderstood, carbohydrates are the body's primary energy source. Focus on whole grains, fruits, vegetables, and legumes, which offer fiber, vitamins, and minerals.
2. **Proteins**: Essential for building and repairing tissues, proteins should be a part of every meal. Options include lean meats, fish, poultry, dairy products, eggs, and plant-based sources like beans and lentils.
3. **Fats**: Healthy fats in avocados, nuts, seeds, olive oil, and fatty fish support brain health, hormone production, and cell

structure. Opt for unsaturated fats while limiting saturated and trans fats.
4. Micronutrients: Vitamins and Minerals

Carbohydrates: Often misunderstood, carbohydrates are the body's primary energy source. Focus on whole grains, fruits, vegetables, and legumes, which offer fiber, vitamins, and minerals.
Proteins: Essential for building and repairing tissues, proteins should be a part of every meal. Options include lean meats, fish, poultry, dairy products, eggs, and plant-based sources like beans and lentils.
Fats: Healthy fats in avocados, nuts, seeds, olive oil, and fatty fish support brain health, hormone production, and cell structure. Opt for unsaturated fats while limiting saturated and trans fats.

Hydration: Water plays a crucial role in every bodily function. Staying well-hydrated aids digestion, nutrient absorption, and waste elimination and can significantly impact your energy levels and physical performance.

The Importance of a Balanced Diet
Weight Management: Proper nutrition helps regulate body weight by providing satiety, stabilizing blood sugar levels, and improving metabolic function.
Disease Prevention: Scientific research has shown that a diet that includes abundant fruits, vegetables, whole grains, and lean proteins can significantly reduce the risk of chronic diseases such as heart disease, diabetes, and certain cancers.
Energy and Well-being: Balanced meals ensure steady energy levels throughout the day, enhancing your ability to engage in somatic practices and maintain overall vitality.

Connecting Nutrition to Somatic Practice
As we delve deeper into "5.2 Foods That Support Somatic Practice," the connection between what we eat and how we move becomes evident. Nutrition directly impacts our **energy levels**, **recovery rates**, and **mental clarity**—crucial for a mindful, effective somatic practice. By adopting nutritional habits that align

with our physical activities, we create a synergistic effect that enhances our bodily health and somatic experience.

Incorporating basic nutrition principles into your daily life lays the groundwork for a holistic approach to well-being, where mindful eating becomes as integral to your health as mindful movement. By understanding and applying these principles, you set the stage for a journey towards harmonized physical and emotional health, where each meal supports your somatic journey, and your dietary choices nourish every movement.

5.2 Foods That Support Somatic Practice

The foods we consume are pivotal in harmonizing physical and emotional well-being, especially when aligned with somatic practices. "5.2 Foods That Support Somatic Practice" delves into the nutritional choices that can significantly enhance your energy levels, flexibility, and recovery, ensuring your body is optimally nourished to support the demands of bodily exercises.

Foods to Enhance Energy: For optimal energy during physical activity, consume complex carbs and whole grains like oats, quinoa, and brown rice. These foods offer a steady release of energy, avoiding spikes and dips in blood sugar levels. Pairing carbohydrates with proteins, such as nuts, seeds, or lean meats, can further stabilize energy levels and keep you satiated, ensuring you have the stamina for your exercises.

Supporting Flexibility with Nutrition: While flexibility is often associated with physical practice, certain nutrients can support the health of your connective tissues, contributing to overall flexibility. Omega-3 fatty acids in fatty fish, flaxseeds, and walnuts help maintain joint health and reduce inflammation, potentially easing movement. Vitamin C-rich foods like citrus fruits, berries, and peppers support collagen production, which is crucial for the strength and elasticity of muscles and tendons.

Nutrition for Optimal Recovery: Post-exercise recovery is as much about what you eat as it is about rest. Protein is an essential nutrient crucial in repairing and building muscle tissues; incorporating lean protein sources such as chicken, tofu, or legumes after your somatic practice can aid muscle recovery. Antioxidant-rich foods, like dark leafy greens, berries, and sweet potatoes, help combat oxidative stress and inflammation in the body, speeding up the recovery process. Additionally, staying hydrated is crucial. Did you know that water is vital for your body's optimal functioning? It supports every metabolic function and nutrient transfer, leading to efficient recovery. So, stay hydrated throughout the day to keep your body in shape!

Magnesium and Muscle Health: Magnesium plays a vital role in muscle function and relaxation, making it an essential mineral for anyone engaged in somatic exercises. Magnesium-rich foods include spinach, pumpkin seeds, and avocados. Incorporating these into your diet can help reduce muscle cramps and improve muscular health and flexibility.

The Role of Electrolytes: Electrolytes, including sodium, potassium, and calcium, are vital for muscle function and fluid balance. Incorporating foods like bananas, sweet potatoes, and dairy products in your diet can effectively replenish the electrolytes lost during exercise, thus aiding in proper hydration and preventing muscle cramps caused by sweating.

As we progress to "5.3 Integrating Nutrition with Somatic Exercises," the interplay between what we eat and how we move becomes increasingly apparent. The right nutritional choices can profoundly impact our ability to engage fully in somatic practices, influencing our energy levels, flexibility, recovery, and overall well-being. This holistic approach underscores the importance of viewing food as fuel and a vital component of our physical and emotional health journey. By aligning our dietary choices with our somatic practices, we create a synergistic effect that amplifies both benefits, leading to a more balanced, healthy, and harmonious life.

Embarking on a nutrition journey, especially with the goal of weight loss, is a commendable but complex process that requires more than just determination and information; it necessitates personalized guidance. Every individual's body is unique, with specific needs, challenges, and goals. Therefore, consulting a professional in the field is crucial. These experts can provide tailored advice, ensuring your diet plan is balanced, sustainable, and conducive to your health. They can help you navigate dietary choices, understand portion control, and integrate nutrition into your lifestyle in a way that supports not just weight loss but overall well-being. Seeking professional guidance ensures your journey is both effective and safe, laying a solid foundation for long-term success.

5.3 Integrating Nutrition with Somatic Exercises

Integrating nutrition with somatic exercises represents a holistic approach to well-being that transcends the boundaries of physical activity alone. In "5.3 Integrating Nutrition with Somatic Exercises," we explore how the synergy between what you eat and how you move can significantly enhance your health, energy levels, and overall effectiveness of your somatic practice. This integration is pivotal as you progress towards "Chapter 6: A 30-Day Somatic Exercise Plan for Weight Loss," where a balanced approach to nutrition and physical activity becomes the cornerstone of achieving sustainable weight loss and enhanced well-being.

Harmonizing Nutrition and Movement

Fusing mindful eating with somatic exercises is not just about choosing the right foods; it's about aligning your nutritional intake with the demands and benefits of your physical practice. This alignment ensures that your body is optimally fueled and nourished, facilitating a deeper connection with your somatic experience and supporting your body's natural healing and strengthening processes.

Pre-Exercise Nutrition: Fueling your body with the right nutrients before engaging in somatic exercises can significantly impact your performance and energy levels. A small, balanced meal or snack with complex carbohydrates and protein about an hour before practice can provide sustained energy. For example, a banana with Greek yogurt and berries offers a mix of quick and slow-releasing energy.

Hydration: Hydration is key to effective somatic practice. Drinking water before, during, and after your exercises ensures that your muscles are well-hydrated, which is crucial for flexibility, strength, and recovery. Incorporating electrolyte-rich foods or drinks post-exercise can also help replenish any minerals lost through sweat.

Post-Exercise Recovery: After somatic exercises, your focus should shift to recovery. Consuming foods rich in protein and carbohydrates helps repair and rebuild muscle tissues and restore energy reserves. A smoothie with protein powder, spinach, and a piece of fruit, or a bowl of quinoa with mixed vegetables and lean protein, are excellent choices to aid recovery.

Anti-Inflammatory Foods: Somatic exercises often work to release tension and reduce inflammation in the body. Complementing this with an anti-inflammatory diet — rich in omega-3 fatty acids, antioxidants, and phytonutrients — can amplify the benefits. Foods like salmon, walnuts, flaxseeds, turmeric, berries, and leafy greens can support the body's natural inflammation response, enhancing flexibility and reducing pain.

Consistency and Mindfulness: Just as somatic exercises promote awareness and intentionality in movement, integrating nutrition requires a mindful approach to eating. Choosing whole, nutrient-dense foods and eating in a relaxed environment can support digestion and absorption of nutrients and enhance your somatic practice by listening to your body's hunger and fullness cues.

Integrating nutrition with somatic exercises becomes a practical guide for creating a balanced, sustainable approach to weight loss and health. This comprehensive strategy ensures that as you work towards physical goals, you also nourish your body and mind, laying the foundation for lasting change and a deeper connection to your well-being.

Chapter 6: A 4-Week Somatic Exercise Plan

6.1 Setting Realistic Goals:

Establishing achievable objectives is crucial for maintaining motivation, tracking progress, and, ultimately, realizing the changes you wish to see in your physical and emotional well-being. This section provides a blueprint for setting practical, attainable goals that resonate with your aspirations and lifestyle, laying a solid foundation as you progress towards "6.2 Weekly Plans with Daily Exercises."

Understanding Realistic Goal Setting

Realistic goal setting involves acknowledging your current physical condition, lifestyle, and time constraints, then determining what you can feasibly achieve within a 30-day timeframe. It's about balance — pushing yourself to grow while setting targets that are within reach to avoid discouragement.

Assess Your Starting Point: Take an honest look at your current physical health, activity level, and dietary habits. Understanding where you are starting from helps tailor your goals to be both challenging and achievable.

Define Clear, Measurable Objectives: Goals should be specific and measurable. Instead of aiming to "lose weight," specify an amount, such as "lose 5 pounds in 30 days." Incorporate somatic practice goals, like "practice somatic exercises for 20 minutes daily," to ensure your objectives cover weight loss and holistic well-being.

Incorporate Short-term Milestones: Breaking down your main goal into smaller, weekly milestones can make the journey more manageable and provide frequent opportunities for celebration. For instance, aim for a specific number of somatic sessions each week or a small, consistent dietary change.

Be Flexible and Kind to Yourself: Recognize that progress is not always linear. There may be days when you feel more energized, and your body needs rest. Adjusting your goals based on feelings is not a setback but a part of mindful practice and self-care.

Seek Balance in Nutrition and Movement: Your goals should reflect a balanced approach to weight loss, combining somatic exercises with mindful eating practices. This holistic view ensures that your objectives support overall health, not just a number on the scale.

Visualize Success: Visualizing yourself and achieving goals regularly can boost motivation and commitment.

Linking Goals to Actions

With your realistic goals set, the transition to "6.2 Weekly Plans with Daily Exercises" becomes a journey of action. This next section will outline a structured plan that aligns with your established objectives, providing daily exercises and nutritional advice to guide you toward your goals. Each week's program is designed to build on the previous one, gradually intensifying your practice to support sustainable weight loss and enhance your bodily experience.

Creating achievable goals is the first step toward a challenging and transformative journey. It's about more than just weight loss; it's about cultivating a lifestyle that harmonizes physical activity, nutrition, and mindfulness for lasting well-being. As you progress through this 30-day plan, remember that each step moves towards a healthier, more balanced you, no matter how small.

6.2 Weekly Plans with Daily Exercises:

To ensure a progressive and incremental approach to the 30-day plan, we will structure the weekly plans into training blocks that gradually increase in difficulty. This structure will incorporate more repetitions, advanced variations of exercises, and deeper mindfulness practices to align with enhancing physical capabilities and nutritional optimization. The aim is to create a balanced, comprehensive program that evolves with your growing strength, flexibility, and emotional resilience.

Week 1: Foundation and Mind-Body Connection
- **Focus**: Establish a baseline of somatic exercises emphasizing form and breath. Introduce basic mindfulness practices and foundational nutritional habits.
- **Somatic Exercises**: Pelvic Clocks, Cat-Cow Stretches (Basic Form).
- **Mindfulness Practices**: Daily 5-minute breath-focused meditation gratitude journaling.
- **Nutritional Advice**: Hydration focus, balanced breakfasts.

Week 2: Building Strength and Flexibility
- **Focus**: Increase the repetitions of week one exercises and introduce new exercises to build strength, particularly in the core and lower body, while continuing to enhance flexibility.
- **Somatic Exercises**: Increase repetitions of Pelvic Clocks and Cat-Cow Stretches and introduce Rolling Bridges and Standing Pelvic Tilts.
- **Mindfulness Practices**: Extend meditation to 10 minutes and introduce body scanning.
- **Nutritional Advice**: Emphasis on protein for muscle repair, introduction of omega-3-rich foods for recovery.

Week 3: Deepening Practice and Enhancing Endurance
- **Focus**: Introduce variations of existing exercises to deepen the practice. Increase the duration and complexity of mindfulness practices. Nutritionally, focus on foods that support endurance and recovery.
- **Somatic Exercises**: Add variations to Rolling Bridges (e.g., single-leg), integrate gentle twists for spinal mobility, and increase overall repetitions.

- **Mindfulness Practices**: Walking meditation, mindful eating practices.
- **Nutritional Advice**: Focus on complex carbohydrates for sustained energy and antioxidant-rich foods for inflammation.

Week 4: Integration and Advanced Practices
- **Focus**: Combine exercises into longer sequences for a comprehensive practice, incorporating advanced variations and increased repetitions. Deepen mindfulness practices and refine nutritional habits.
- **Somatic Exercises**: Sequence combining all previous exercises with added complexity (e.g., dynamic Cat-Cow into Rolling Bridge), introduce side planks for core stability.
- **Mindfulness Practices**: Engage in guided meditation integrating mind-body practices, journal reflections on progress, and insights.
- **Nutritional Advice**: Balanced approach focusing on meal timing around exercises, hydration, and incorporating a variety of nutrients to support holistic health.

This incremental approach ensures a continuous challenge and engagement for the body and mind, encouraging growth, adaptation, and a deeper understanding of the interconnectedness between physical activity, mindfulness, and nutrition. Each week builds upon the last, ensuring a cohesive and comprehensive journey towards achieving your weight loss and wellness goals.

Week 1: Foundation and Mind-Body Connection

Week 1 will focus on establishing a solid somatic movement and mindfulness base. This week, the exercises are designed to help you become aware of your body's signals and how they connect to your sense of well-being. The goal is to perform these exercises with attention to form and breath, allowing for a gentle introduction to the practice.

Let's start the somatic exercises of week 1!

Pelvic Clocks

This exercise improves pelvic awareness and control, helping to establish a connection with your core.

How to Perform: Please Lie flat on your back with your knees bent and feet on the ground. Imagine a clock on your pelvis with 12 o'clock towards your head and 6 o'clock towards your feet. Gently rock your pelvis towards each number on the clock.

Repetitions: Perform this movement for 3 minutes, making sure to move slowly and with control.

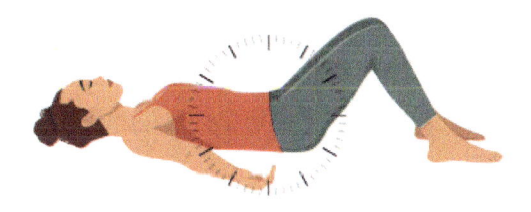

Cat-Cow Stretches (Basic Form)

Cat-cow stretches are fundamental for spinal flexibility and core engagement.

How to Perform: Start on your hands and knees in a tabletop position. Begin in a tabletop position with your hands and knees on the ground. Ensure your wrists are positioned directly beneath your shoulders and your knees are placed directly under your hips. As you inhale, draw your chest forward and, at the same time, drop your belly towards the floor. Lift your head and tailbone towards the ceiling, creating an arch in your spine (Cow pose). As you exhale, round your spine towards the ceiling, pulling your belly button towards your spine. Tuck your chin to your chest and let your head hang heavy (Cat pose). Repeat this movement, flowing back and forth between Cow and Cat poses with each inhale and exhale, feeling the stretch in your back and neck.

Repetitions: Complete this sequence for 3 minutes, flowing smoothly between Cat and Cow and synchronizing each movement with your breath.

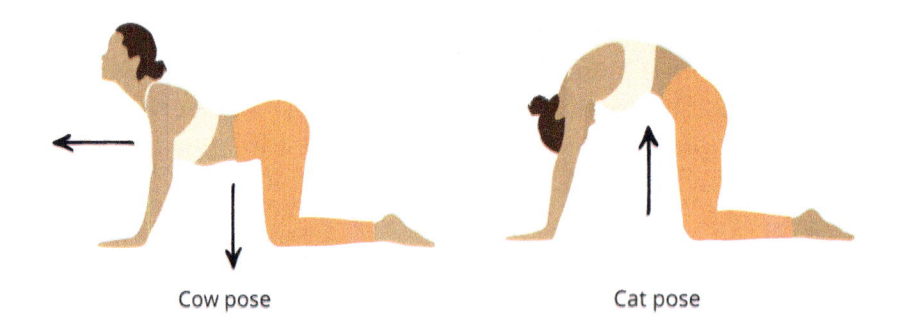

Cow pose

Cat pose

Knee-to-Chest Stretch

This stretch gently releases the lower back and hips, promoting relaxation and lower body awareness.

How to Perform: Lie on your back with both legs extended. Gently draw one knee into your chest, clasping your hands around your shin. If more comfortable, keep the other leg flat on the ground or with a bent knee. Hold the stretch for a few deep breaths, focusing on the release in your lower back and hips, then switch legs.

Repetitions: Alternate legs for 3 minutes, spending approximately 45 seconds on each side with each repetition.

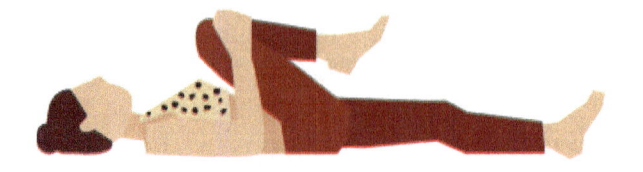

Spinal Twist

Spinal Twists aid spinal mobility and can gently stretch the back muscles, encouraging proper alignment and relaxation.

How to Perform: Remain to lie on your back, and bring your arms out to a T-shape for stability. Keeping your knees bent and together, let them fall gently to one side, keeping your shoulders on the ground. Turn your head in the opposite direction of your knees to complete the twist. After several breaths, return your knees to the center and repeat on the other side.

Repetitions: Hold each twist for 30 seconds to 1 minute on each side, performing the sequence for 3 minutes.

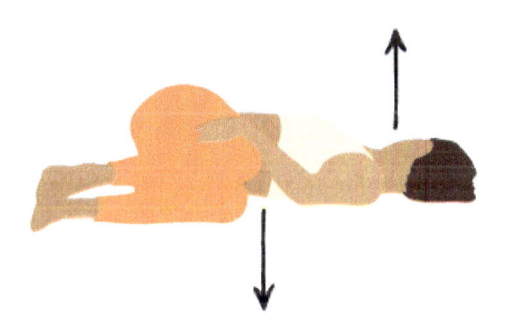

Child's Pose

This resting pose stretches the lower back and hips, calms the brain, and helps relieve stress and fatigue, making it perfect for enhancing the mind-body connection.

How to Perform: From a tabletop position, lower your hips back to rest on your heels, forehead touching the mat, with your arms extended in front of you or by your sides. Breathe deeply in this position, allowing your lower back to relax and stretch naturally.

Duration: Hold for 2-3 minutes, focusing on deep breathing to encourage relaxation and release tension.

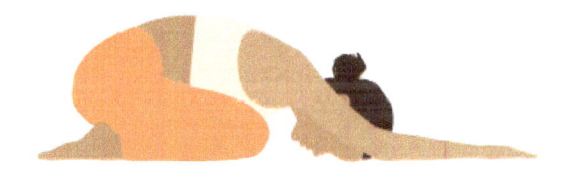

Supine March

Supine marching gently engages the core and stabilizes the pelvis, improving body awareness and effortless core strength.

How to perform: To perform this exercise, you must lie on your back with your knees bent and your arms straight and relaxed along your sides. To succeed best with this exercise. Engaging the core muscles by bringing the belly button toward the spine is important to maintain a neutral spine position. This position ensures proper back alignment and helps avoid unnecessary tension or discomfort. Slowly lower one foot to the floor and then re-establish it in the starting position, alternating legs as if you were marching in place.

Repetitions: Perform this march for 3 minutes, keeping the core engaged to prevent the back from arching.

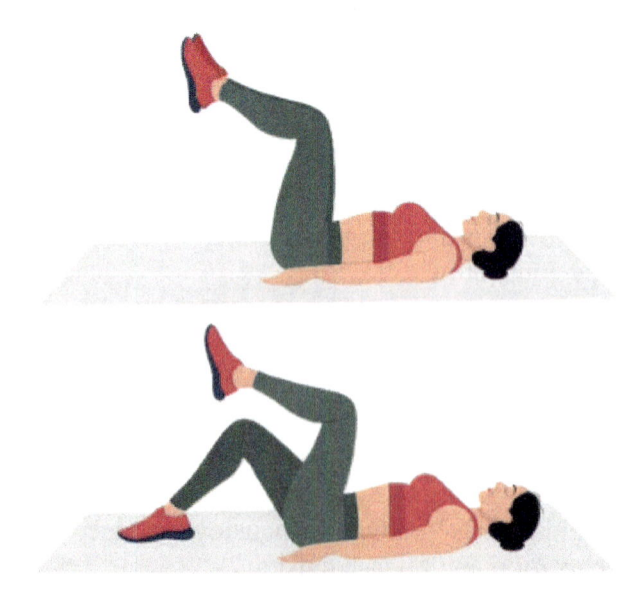

During Week 1, the focus is on quality over quantity. Rather than aiming for many repetitions, concentrate on performing each movement with intention and awareness. Listen to your body and allow the exercises to be meditative, fostering a strong connection between mind and body. This week sets the stage for more complex movements and a deeper somatic experience in the weeks to come.

During this first week, as you lay the groundwork for your somatic journey, nutritional support is as vital as your exercise routine. A focus on hydration and balanced breakfasts sets the stage for energy, recovery, and mental clarity throughout the day.

Hydration Focus
Start your day by hydrating your body. Overnight, you go without water for several hours, so beginning with a glass or two can kick start your hydration. Carrying a water bottle with you throughout the day is recommended as a reminder to drink water regularly. If plain water doesn't appeal to you, infuse it with slices of cucumber, lemon, or berries for a refreshing twist. Proper hydration aids digestion, nutrient absorption, and even muscle flexibility, which is crucial when engaging in somatic exercises.

Balanced Breakfasts
A balanced breakfast is essential as it provides the necessary energy and nutrients to kick-start your day. You are needed to fuel your body for the day ahead. Aim for a combination of complex carbohydrates for sustained energy, proteins for muscle support, and healthy fats for satiety and brain health. A balanced breakfast with essential nutrients such as proteins, carbohydrates, and healthy fats can provide sustained energy throughout the day. For instance, you can have a bowl of oatmeal with almonds and blueberries or a spinach and feta omelet with whole-grain toast. Such meals support your physical activities and help stabilize blood sugar levels, manage appetite and mood, and keep you going all day.

Remember, your chosen foods are as integral to your practice as the exercises. Week 1's nutritional advice is designed to complement your somatic exercises, creating a harmonious blend of movement and nourishment that supports your overall well-being and weight loss goals.

WEEK 1 *Exercises*

PELVIC CLOCKS
3 MINUTES

CAT-COW STRETCHES
3 MINUTES

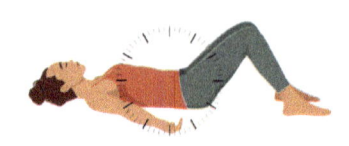

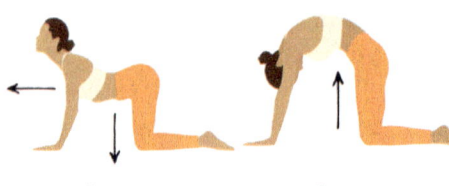

Cow pose   Cat pose

KNEE-TO-CHEST STRETCH
3 MINUTES

SPINAL TWIST
30 SECONDS TO 1 MINUTE ON EACH SIDE
3 MINUTES

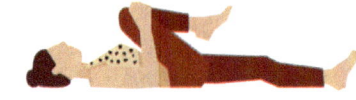

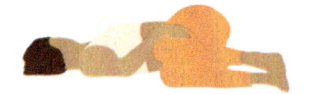

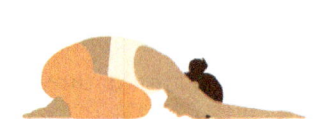

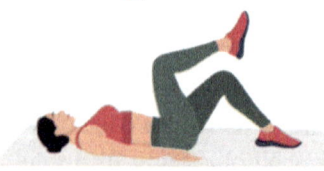

CHILD'S POSE
3 MINUTES

SUPINE MARCH
3 MINUTES

Week 2: Foundation and Mind-Body Connection

For Week 2 of "Building Strength and Flexibility," we will build upon the foundational exercises from Week 1 and incorporate additional movements designed to enhance your strength and flexibility further. This week, you will notice an increase in repetitions and the introduction of new exercises to challenge your body progressively.

Let's start the second week!

Pelvic Clocks

Same exercise as *Week 1* with a slight modification: aiming for a slightly more extensive range of motion as your awareness and control improve.

Repetitions: Practice the exercise for about **5 minutes**

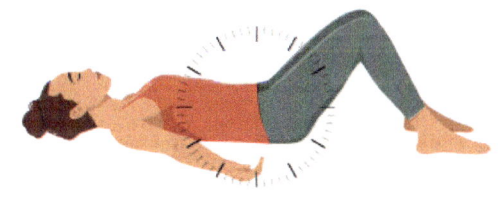

Cat-Cow Stretches

It is the same exercise as *Week 1* with a slight modification: emphasizing fluidity and deeper spinal flexion and extension.

Repetitions: Increase to **5 minutes.**

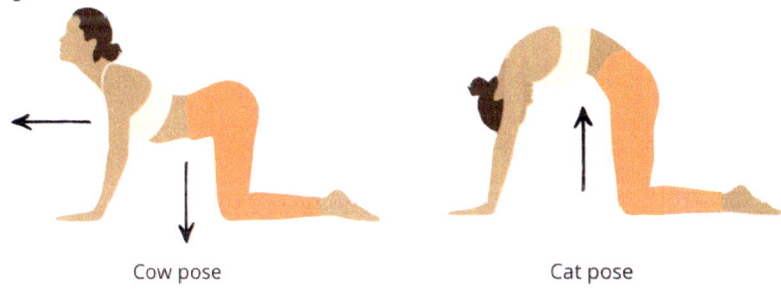

Cow pose   Cat pose

Child's Pose

Same exercise as *Week 1* with the **Duration** modification: Extend this pose to **3-5 minutes**, using deep breaths to enhance the stretch in the lower back and hips.

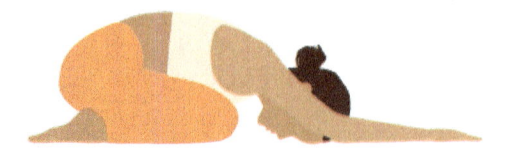

Supine Marching

Same as *Week 1* - slight modification on the:

Repetitions: Perform for **5 minutes**, focusing on keeping your pelvis stable and your core engaged throughout the movement.

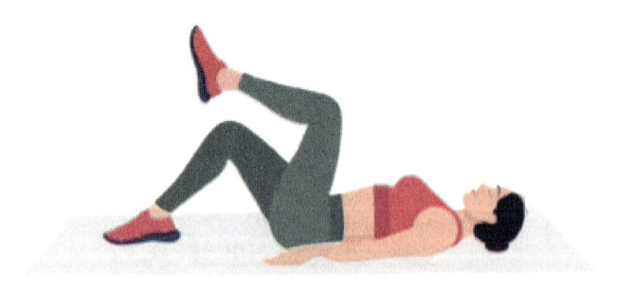

NEW THIS WEEK:

Downward Dog

Description: Strengthens the entire body, focusing on the shoulders, hamstrings, and core.

How to Perform: Begin by positioning yourself on all fours with your hands and knees on the mat. It is essential that the wrists are perfectly below the shoulders and your knees are aligned with your hips. From here, lift your hips up towards the top and push your hands and feet to create an inverted V-shape with your body. Keep your head and neck relaxed, and engage your core to maintain balance. Hold the position for a few breaths, feeling the stretch in your hamstrings and calves. Slowly release and return to the starting position. If you can't keep your legs totally extended, it doesn't matter; you can bend them slightly.

Duration: Hold for 30-60 seconds for 3 sets, resting in Child's Pose in between.

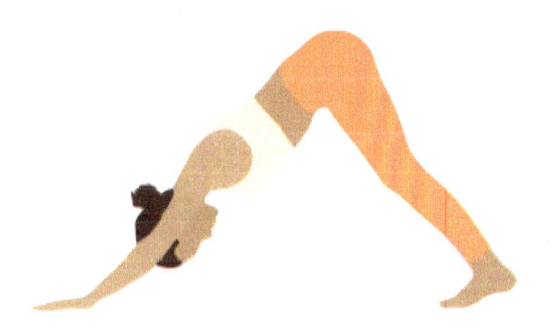

Crescent Lunge Yoga Pose

This dynamic yoga pose engages the quadriceps, opens the hips, and builds lower body strength. It also stretches the hip flexors and encourages good posture and balance.

How to Perform:
Get on your knees on a mat. Bring your left leg back with your foot resting on the mat. Now, bring your right leg to the front and Bend the knee until it forms a 90-degree angle, ensuring it is perfectly above the ankle.
Raise your arms above your head and keep them parallel, with your palms facing each other or touching.
Sink into the lunge to intensify the hip flexor stretch.
Keep your gaze forward or slightly up toward your hands while maintaining a steady breath. Then, switch legs.

Duration: Hold the Crescent Lunge for 30 seconds to 1 minute, then release and switch sides. Repeat for 2-3 sets on each side.

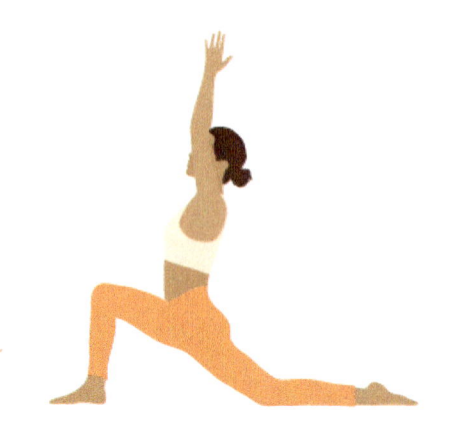

Seated Forward Fold

Good exercise to stretch the hamstrings and lower back, promoting flexibility.

How to Perform: Sit and extend your legs in front of you. Inhale to lengthen the spine, and hinge at the hips to fold forward as you exhale. Reach towards your feet, or place your hands on the ground beside your legs.

Duration: Hold for 1-2 minutes, gently deepening the stretch with each exhale.

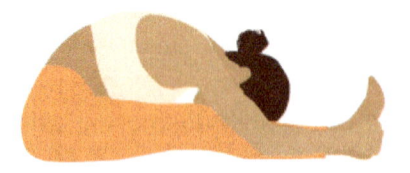

Seated Spinal Twist

Increases spinal mobility and stretches the back muscles.

How to Perform: Sit on the edge of a sturdy chair or on the floor with your legs crossed, spine high, and shoulders relaxed. Begin by slowly rotating your torso to the right, keeping your hips facing forward to isolate the rotation in your upper body. Let the head follow the torso's movement so the neck remains aligned with the spine.

Begin the twist (seated): Place your right hand on your left knee and your left hand behind your back or on the seat for support. Then, gently return to the center and repeat the movement on the opposite side.

Inhale deeply in the starting position, and as you exhale, deepen into the twist.

Repetitions: Hold for 30 seconds on each side, performing 2 sets.

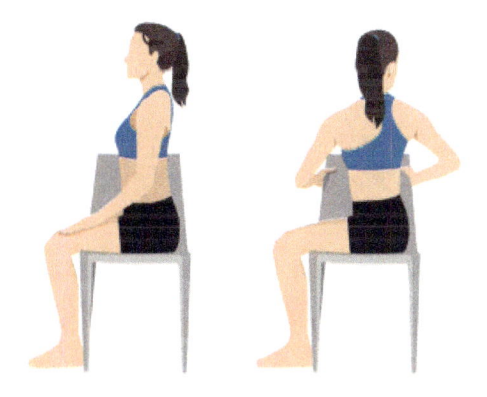

Bridge Pose

Builds lower body strength, particularly in the glutes and hamstrings, and engages the core.

How to Perform: Start by lying down on your back. Bend your knees and ensure that your feet are firmly on the ground. Next, press your feet into the ground and engage your glutes to lift your hips towards the ceiling, creating a bridge-like position with your body. Hold this position for a few seconds before slowly lowering your hips back to the ground. Repeat the exercise for several reps to strengthen your glutes and lower back muscles.

Repetitions: Hold for 30 seconds for 3 sets, focusing on engaging the glutes and core.

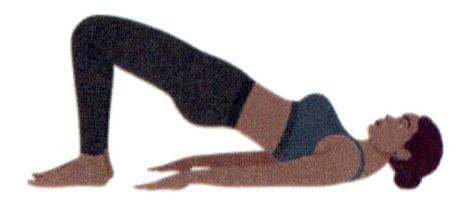

Warrior II

Enhances leg strength, opens the hips, and increases body awareness and balance.

How to Perform: Stand with feet wide apart, turn one foot out, and bend into the knee, extending arms to the sides at shoulder height.

Duration: Hold for 30 seconds to 1 minute on each side, and perform two sets.

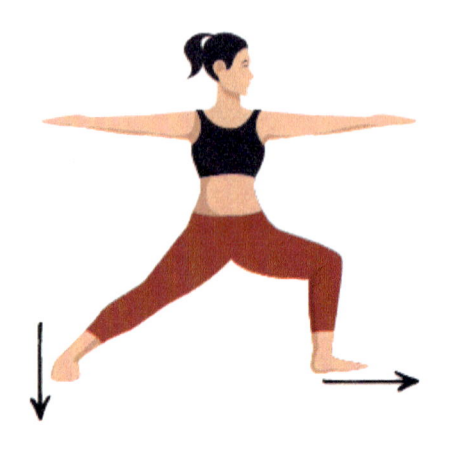

In Week 2, as you engage with these exercises, pay close attention to your body's responses. The increase in repetitions and the introduction of new stretches are designed to challenge your muscles and promote greater flexibility, preparing you for more advanced practices in the upcoming weeks. Remember to practice mindfulness with each movement, keeping your breath steady and your focus on the sensations within your body.

Nutrition advice: In Week 2, as your somatic exercises intensify, supporting your body's need for muscle repair and recovery becomes paramount. This week, we strongly emphasize protein and the introduction of omega-3-rich foods to aid in this process.
Protein is critical in repairing muscle fibers that are worked and stretched during your exercises. Incorporating a variety of proteins into your meals ensures that your muscles receive the essential amino acids they need to recover and strengthen. Consider lean meats, fish, dairy, **legumes**, and plant-based proteins like **quinoa** and **tofu**. Remember to include a protein source in every meal to support continuous muscle repair.

Omega-3 fatty acids, found abundantly in fatty fish like **salmon**, **mackerel**, and **sardines**, as well as in **flaxseeds**, **chia seeds**, and **walnuts**, offer powerful anti-inflammatory benefits. These nutrients are crucial for reducing inflammation that may occur with increased physical activity, aiding in faster recovery and better joint health. Incorporating these foods into your diet supports physical recovery and benefits your overall heart health and cognitive function.

By focusing on protein and omega-3-rich foods this week, you're not just aiding in muscle repair and recovery but investing in your body's long-term health and resilience, ensuring you're nourished and vital for the challenges and progress ahead in your journey.

WEEK 2
Exercises

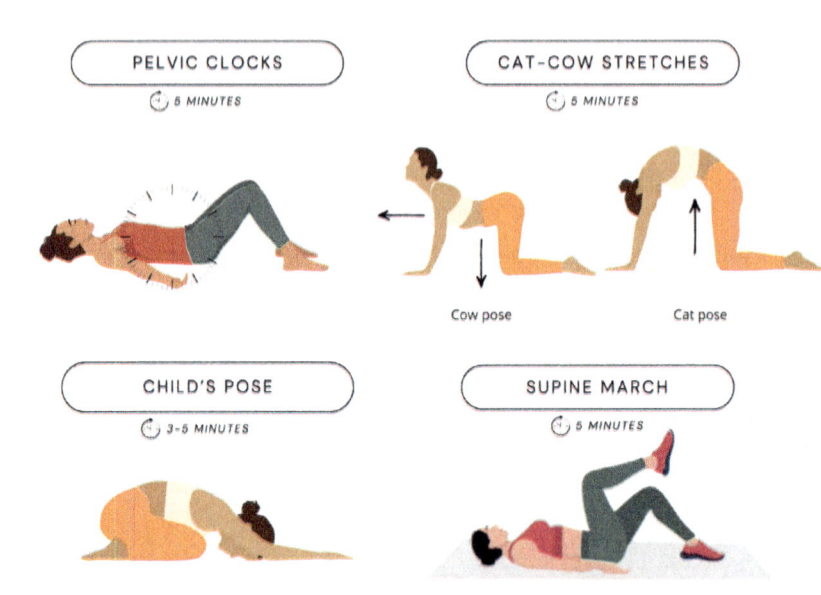

PELVIC CLOCKS
5 MINUTES

CAT-COW STRETCHES
5 MINUTES

Cow pose   Cat pose

CHILD'S POSE
3-5 MINUTES

SUPINE MARCH
5 MINUTES

NEW THIS WEEK

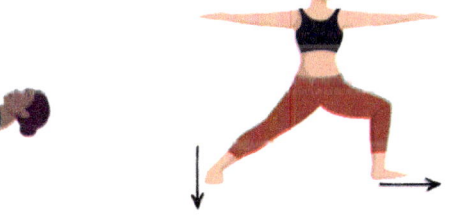

DOWNWARD DOG
30-60 SECONDS FOR 3 SETS

CRESCENT LUNGE YOGA POSE
30 SECONDS TO 1 MINUTE
2-3 SETS EACH SIDE

SEATED FORWARD FOLD
1-2 MINUTES

SEATED SPINAL TWIST
30 SECONDS ON EACH SIDE
2 SETS

BRIDGE POSE
30 SECONDS FOR 3 SETS

WARRIOR II
30 SECONDS TO 1 MINUTE ON EACH SIDE

Week 3: Deepening Practice and Enhancing Endurance

In Week 3, we progress by adding complexity to the movements and increasing the duration of the exercises to build endurance. This week, you will challenge your body further, deepen your mind-body connection, and continue to foster strength and flexibility.

Dynamic Pelvic Clocks

Repetitions: Continue with 5 minutes, adding dynamic movements by lifting the hips slightly off the floor as you circle through the 'hours.'

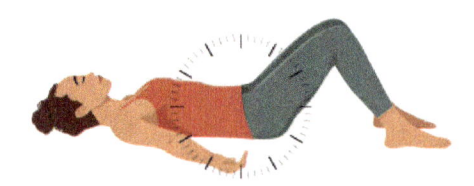

Cat-Cow with Leg Extension

Alternate between Cat and Cow poses, and during the Cow pose, extend one leg back, alternating legs with each repetition.
Repetitions: 5 minutes total.

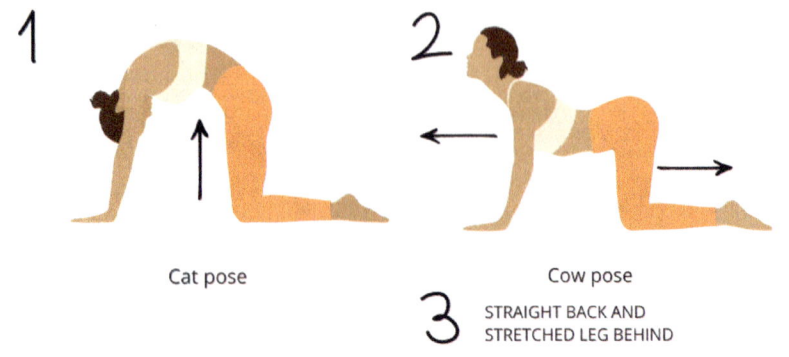

Child's Pose to Extended Puppy Pose

Duration: Transition between poses for 5 minutes, using each inhale to move into the Puppy Pose and exhale to return to the Child's Pose.

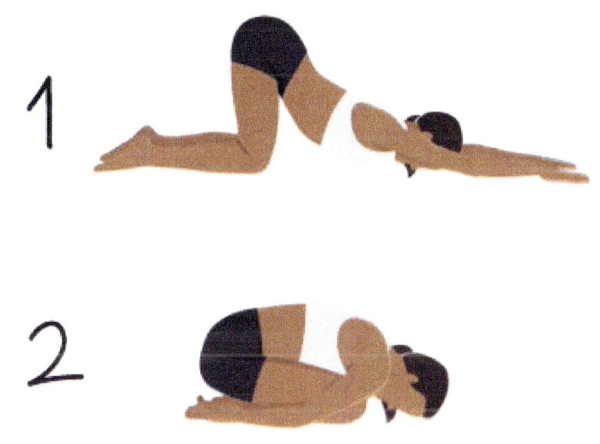

Supine Marching with Arm Movements

Repetitions: Perform for 5 minutes, raising the opposite arm over your head as you lift each leg, keeping the core engaged.

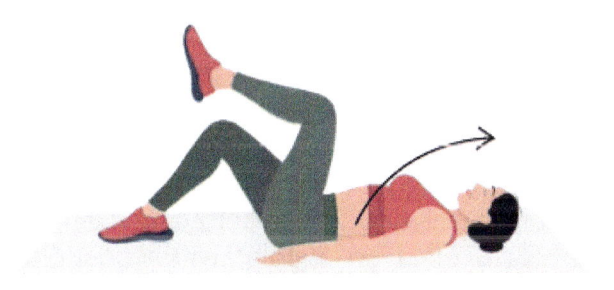

NEW ADDITIONS FOR WEEK 3:

Warrior I to Warrior III Flow

This flow builds lower body strength, improves balance, and engages the core.

How to Perform:

1. **Starting in <u>Warrior I</u> Pose**:

Begin in Warrior I with your right foot forward, knee bent at a 90-degree angle, and your left leg extended behind you, foot flat and angled at about 45 degrees to the front of your mat. Raise your arms overhead, keeping them parallel, shoulders down, and your torso upright.

2. **Transition to <u>Warrior II</u>**

Find Your Focus: Keep your eyes fixed in one spot to help you keep your balance.

Now rotate the pelvis to the right, open the toe of the left foot, extend the left leg well back, making sure the two heels are parallel and the pelvis well open frontally, bend the right knee, and keep the right leg taut and active, having with the right foot rotated to 45 degrees and well adhered to the ground. Feel the weight of the body evenly distributed on the feet.

3. **<u>Warrior III</u> Pose**:

Now, your right leg supports you, with your left leg lifted and extended straight behind you, and your torso and arms grow forward. Your body should form a capital "T" shape. The standing leg's knee can have a slight bend to avoid hyperextension. Focus on lengthening from your back heel through your fingertips and keeping your gaze fixed on a point on the floor to help with balance.

Breath and Hold: Maintain steady, even breaths. Holding Warrior III for 30 seconds to a minute, then carefully reverse the movement to return to Warrior I before switching sides (leg)

It is *important* to do the whole transition with the same leg in front, first the right, then the left

Repetitions: Flow between Warrior I and Warrior III for 1 minute, then switch sides. Perform 2-3 sets on each side.

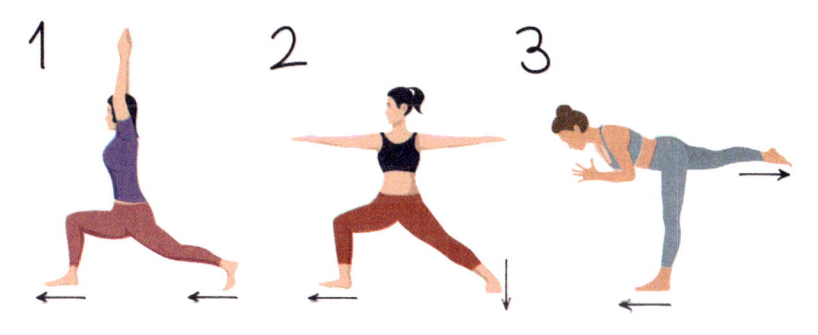

Crescent Lunge with Twist

Adds a rotational challenge to the Crescent Lunge to enhance core strength and spinal flexibility.

How to Perform: From Crescent Lunge, bring your hands into a prayer position at your chest, then rotate your torso and hook your opposite elbow outside your bent knee. Hold the twist and maintain balance.

Duration: Hold the twist for 30 seconds on each side, performing 2-3 sets.

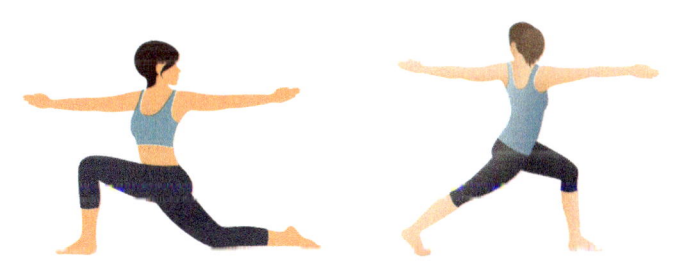

Standing Figure Four Stretch

Stretches the glutes and hips, promoting flexibility and balance.

How to Perform: Stand and cross one ankle over the opposite thigh just above the knee, creating a '4' shape. Bend your standing knee slightly and sit back as if sitting in a chair, keeping your chest lifted.

Duration: Hold for 30 seconds to 1 minute on each side, performing 2-3 sets.

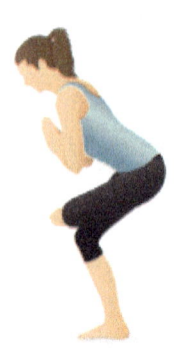

Plank Pose

Strengthens the core, shoulders, and arms and enhances endurance.

How to Perform: From a push-up position, hold your body straight from your heels to your head, hands directly under your shoulders and core engaged.

Duration: Hold for 30 seconds to 1 minute, working up to longer durations. Perform 2-3 sets.

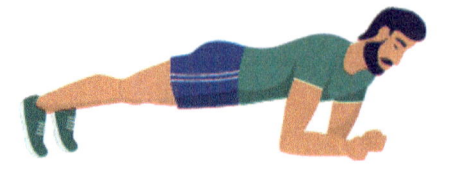

Boat Pose

Strengthens the core, especially the deep abdominal muscles, and improves balance.

How to Perform: Sit flat on the floor with your knees bent. Lean back slightly and lift your feet, extending your arms forward. Balance on your sit bones, keeping your spine straight.

Duration: Hold for 20-30 seconds, performing 2-3 sets.

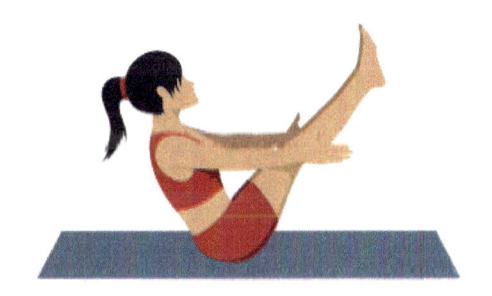

Seated Wide-Legged Forward Fold

Enhances flexibility in the hamstrings and lower back.

How to Perform: Sit with legs wide apart, inhale to lengthen the spine, and exhale as you hinge at the hips to fold forward, walking your hands out in front of you.

Duration: Hold for 2-3 minutes, gradually deepening the stretch.

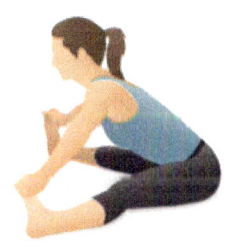

In Week 3, focus on performing these exercises with control and precision, ensuring that you maintain a connection with your body throughout each movement. This week is about pushing your limits while still honoring your body's feedback, fostering endurance and resilience in both your physical and somatic practices.

Nutritional advice: In Week 3, as your practice deepens and endurance is increasingly challenged, your nutritional focus shifts towards fueling your body with sustained energy and supporting recovery with antioxidant-rich foods. This nutritional strategy complements the intensification of your somatic exercises and mindfulness practices.

Complex Carbohydrates for Sustained Energy: Complex carbohydrates are vital this week for maintaining energy levels through more extended and demanding sessions. Foods like whole grains (**brown rice, quinoa,** and **oats**), starchy vegetables (**sweet potatoes** and **squash**), and legumes (**beans** and **lentils**) are excellent sources. These carbohydrates are broken down and absorbed slowly, providing a steady release of energy and keeping you fueled and focused throughout your practice and daily activities.

Antioxidant-Rich Foods for Inflammation: Incorporate various antioxidant-rich foods into your diet to combat potential inflammation and aid in recovery. **Berries, dark leafy greens, nuts, and seeds contain vitamins, minerals**, and antioxidants that help neutralize free radicals and reduce inflammation. Foods high in omega-3 fatty acids, such as flaxseeds, chia seeds, and walnuts, also offer anti-inflammatory benefits. Spices like turmeric and ginger can also be added to meals for an extra anti-inflammatory boost.

Combining complex carbohydrates with antioxidant-rich foods ensures your body has the necessary fuel and protection to support increased physical activity and recovery. This balanced approach to nutrition not only aids in your somatic practice but also contributes to overall health and well-being, enabling you to tackle the challenges of Week 3 with energy and resilience.

WEEK 3
Exercises

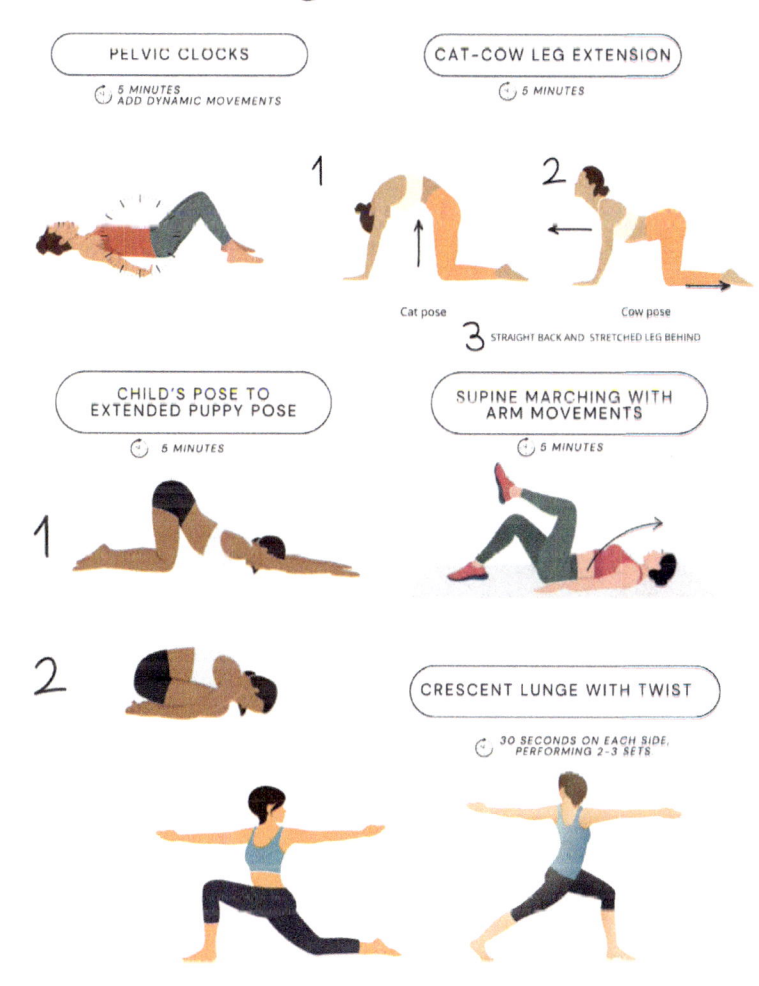

PELVIC CLOCKS
⏱ 5 MINUTES
ADD DYNAMIC MOVEMENTS

CAT-COW LEG EXTENSION
⏱ 5 MINUTES

1 Cat pose

2 Cow pose

3 STRAIGHT BACK AND STRETCHED LEG BEHIND

CHILD'S POSE TO EXTENDED PUPPY POSE
⏱ 5 MINUTES

1

2

SUPINE MARCHING WITH ARM MOVEMENTS
⏱ 5 MINUTES

CRESCENT LUNGE WITH TWIST
⏱ 30 SECONDS ON EACH SIDE, PERFORMING 2-3 SETS

NEW THIS WEEK

WARRIOR I TO WARRIOR III FLOW
1-2 1 MINUTE FOR LEG
2-3 SETS ON EACH SIDE

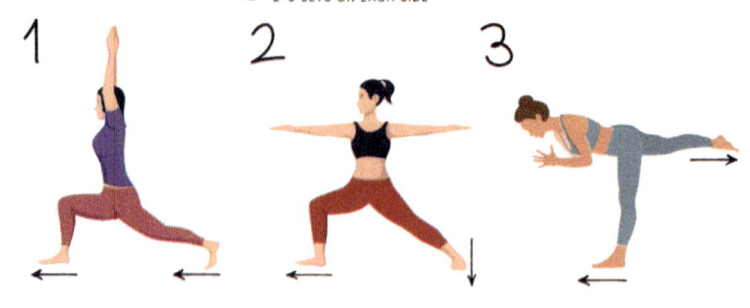

STANDING FIGURE FOUR STRETCH
30 SECONDS TO 1 MINUTE ON EACH SIDE, 2-3 SETS

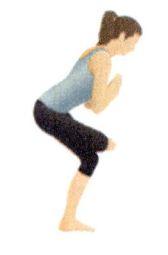

PLANK POSE
30 SECONDS TO 1 MINUTE, 2-3 SETS

BOAT POSE
20-30 SECONDS, 2-3 SETS

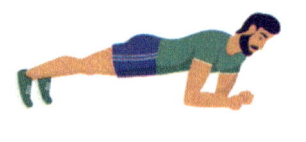

SEATED WIDE-LEGGED FORWARD FOLD
2-3 MINUTES

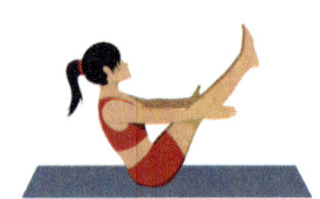

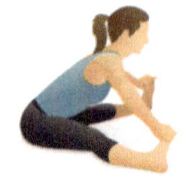

Week 4: Integration and Advanced Practices

In Week 4, we are focusing on consolidating the exercises learned in the previous weeks and introducing advanced variations to challenge your body further and solidify the mind-body connection. This week's exercises are designed to integrate the strength, flexibility, and mindfulness you have developed into a cohesive practice that enhances endurance and prepares you for continued progress beyond the 30-day plan.

Dynamic Cat-Cow with Balancing

Repetitions: 5 minutes total. Extend the opposite arm and leg during the Cow pose, balancing and breathing before switching sides.

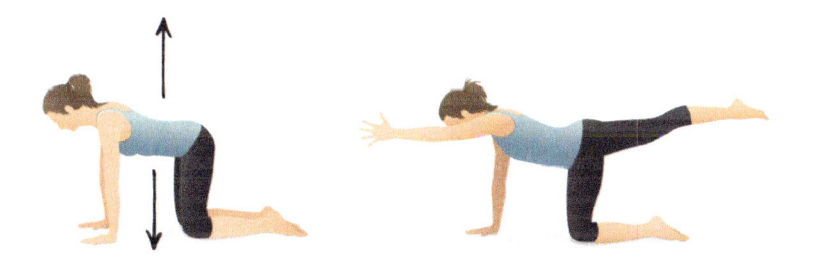

Advanced Pelvic Clocks with Leg Lifts

Repetitions: 5 minutes, incorporating leg lifts while performing pelvic clocks to engage the core and lower body further.

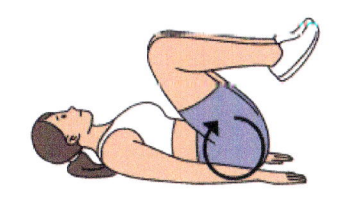

Extended Child's Pose to Downward Dog Flow

Duration: Flow between these poses for 5 minutes, focusing on the transition and alignment in each pose.

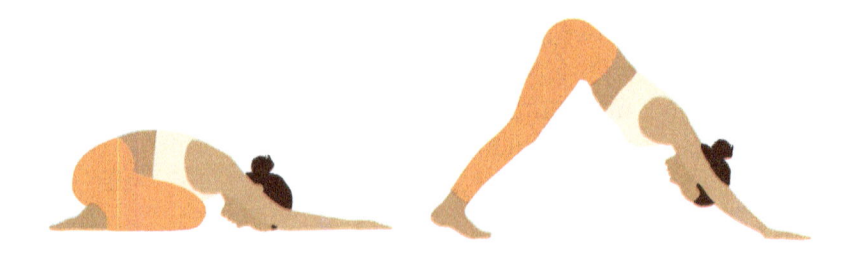

Supine Twists with Leg Extension

Repetitions: Lie on your back, extend one leg up, and gently twist across the body, holding for 30 seconds per side. Perform 3 sets.

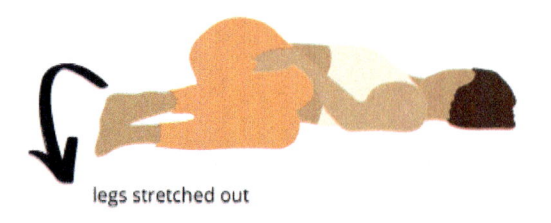

legs stretched out

NEW ADDITIONS FOR WEEK 4

Handstand Prep or Wall Planks

Prepares the body for handstands, building upper body strength and core stability.

How to Perform: Begin in Downward Dog with feet against a wall. Walk your feet up the wall until your body is as vertical as possible, resembling a handstand. Keep your core tight and push through your shoulders.

Duration: Hold for 15-30 seconds, gradually increasing the time as you gain strength. Perform 2-3 sets.

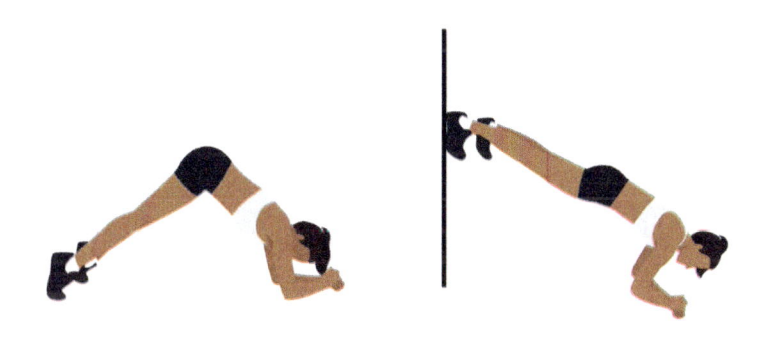

Pigeon Pose

Opens the hips and stretches the hip flexors and glutes, essential for flexibility and recovery.

How to Perform: From Downward Dog, bring one knee forward to the wrist and extend the other leg back. Square your hips and fold forward for a deeper stretch.

Duration: Hold for 2-3 minutes on each side, breathing deeply to encourage relaxation and hip opening.

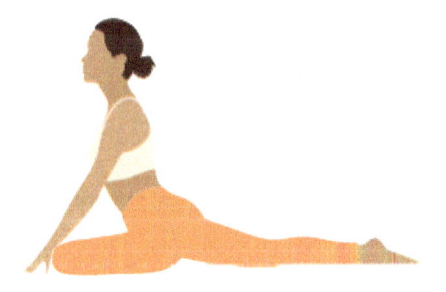

Standing Leg Raises

Strengthens the core, improves balance, and enhances leg flexibility.

How to Perform: Stand on one leg and raise the other leg to the front, side, and back, keeping the core engaged and the movements controlled.

Repetitions: Perform 10-15 leg raises in each direction per leg. Complete 2-3 sets.

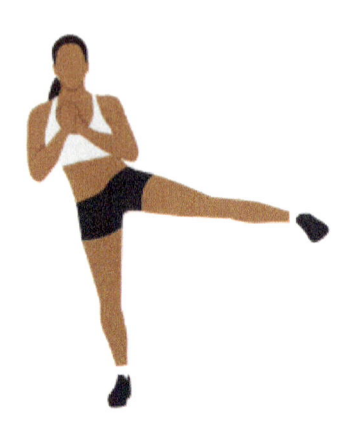

Crow Pose

Builds arm strength, wrist stability, and core engagement.

How to Perform: From a squat, place your hands on the floor, knees resting on your upper arms. Shift your weight forward, lifting your feet off the ground and balancing on your hands.

Duration: Hold for as long as you can maintain form, aiming for 20-30 seconds. Perform 2-3 attempts.

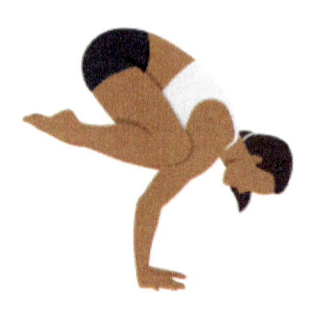

Warrior III

Challenges balance and strengthens the entire body, emphasizing the core and standing leg.

How to Perform: From a standing position, lean forward, lift one leg behind you, and extend your arms forward, creating a 'T' shape with your body.

Duration: Hold for 30-60 seconds on each side. Perform 2-3 sets.

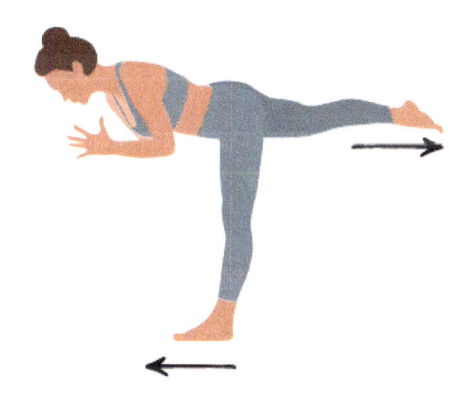

Seated Meditation with Deep Breathing

Duration: After your physical practice, sit for a 10-minute meditation, focusing on deep, diaphragmatic breaths to integrate the benefits of your somatic practice and center your mind.

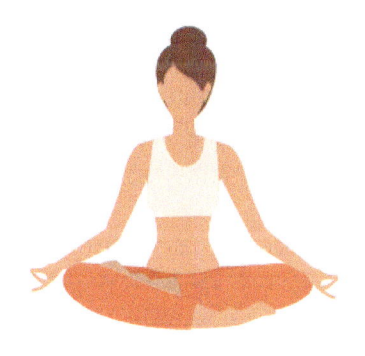

Week 4 brings together all the elements of your 30-day journey, challenging you to maintain focus, deepen your practice, and solidify the habits you've developed. This week is about integration, where each exercise is performed not just for physical benefit but as a part of a holistic approach to well-being that you can carry into your daily life.

Nutritional Advice: In Week 4, as you integrate and advance your practices, the nutritional focus shifts towards a balanced approach that encompasses meal timing around exercises, consistent hydration, and a diverse intake of nutrients. This holistic nutritional strategy is designed to optimize your energy, recovery, and overall health, supporting the culmination of your efforts in this transformative journey.

Meal Timing Around Exercises: Maximizing energy levels during your somatic exercises and enhancing recovery afterward by being mindful of when you eat is crucial. A small, easily digestible snack rich in carbohydrates and protein about 30 to 60 minutes before your practice can provide the necessary fuel without discomfort. Examples include a banana with almond butter or a small serving of Greek yogurt with berries. Following your exercise, aim to consume a balanced meal within two hours to support muscle repair and replenish energy stores. This meal should include a mix of carbohydrates, protein, and healthy fats, such as grilled chicken, quinoa, and avocado salad.

Hydration: Proper hydration is essential, especially as your practice intensity peaks. Aim to drink water consistently throughout the day, not just during exercise sessions. Hydrating foods like cucumbers, watermelon, and oranges can also contribute to your overall fluid intake, aiding in joint lubrication, nutrient transportation, and body temperature regulation.

Incorporating a Variety of Nutrients: This week, focus on diversifying your nutrient intake to support the holistic health benefits of your somatic and mindful practices. Ensure your diet includes various vitamins and minerals by consuming **fruits**, **vegetables**, **whole grains**, **lean proteins**, and **healthy fats**. Each color represents different nutrients, so the more varied your plate, the broader the benefits you'll receive. Foods rich in magnesium, such as spinach, nuts, and seeds, can aid muscle relaxation and recovery, while foods high in calcium, like dairy products and leafy greens, support bone health.

By adopting a balanced nutritional approach in Week 4, focusing on meal timing, hydration, and nutrient diversity, you're not just fueling your body for the present; you're establishing habits that promote long-term health and vitality. This comprehensive strategy ensures you're well-equipped to continue your journey beyond this program with the nutritional foundation necessary to support a life of wellness and harmony.

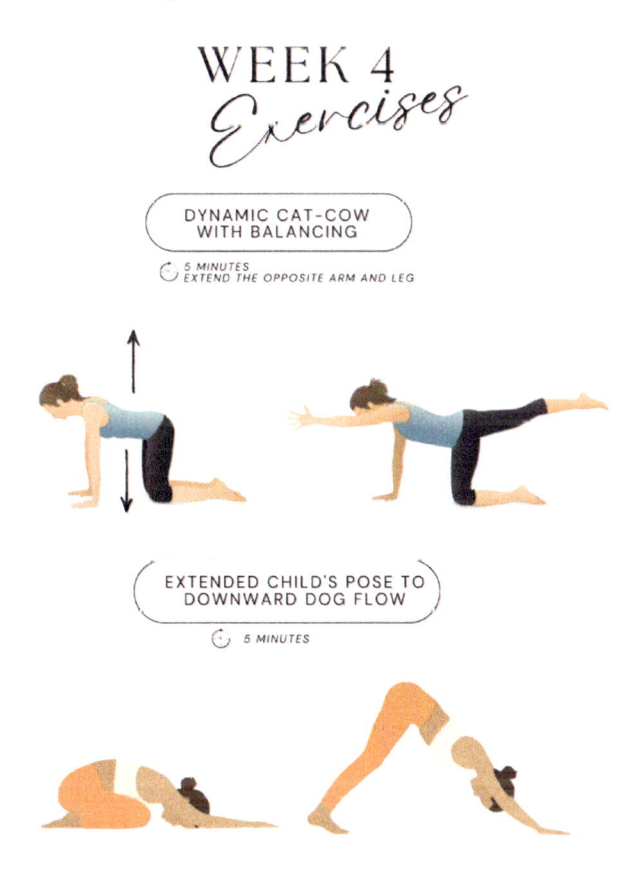

WEEK 4 Exercises

DYNAMIC CAT-COW WITH BALANCING

5 MINUTES
EXTEND THE OPPOSITE ARM AND LEG

EXTENDED CHILD'S POSE TO DOWNWARD DOG FLOW

5 MINUTES

SUPINE TWISTS WITH LEG EXTENSION	ADVANCED PELVIC CLOCKS WITH LEG LIFTS
30 SECONDS PER SIDE, 3 SETS	5 MINUTES

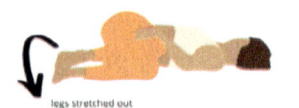

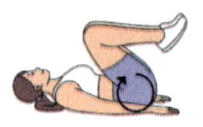

NEW THIS WEEK

HANDSTAND PREP OR WALL PLANKS

15-30 SECONDS, 2-3 SETS.

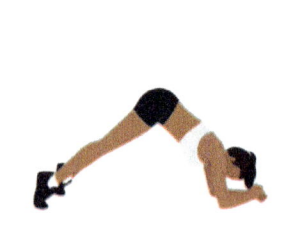

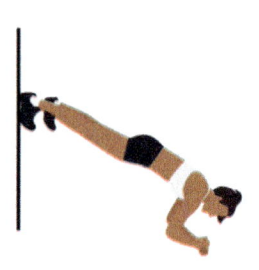

PIGEON POSE	STANDING LEG RAISES
2-3 MINUTES ON EACH SIDE	10-15 LEG RAISES IN EACH DIRECTION PER LEG, 2-3 SETS

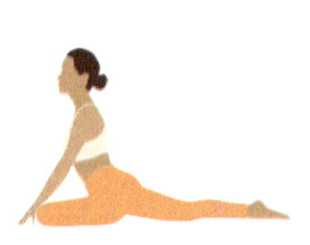

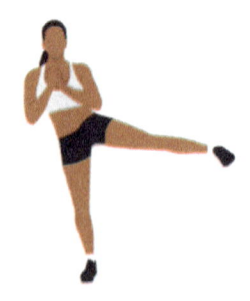

CROW POSE

⏱ 20-30 SECONDS, 2-3 ATTEMPTS

WARRIOR III

⏱ 30-60 SECONDS ON EACH SIDE. 2-3 SETS.

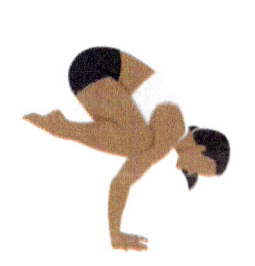

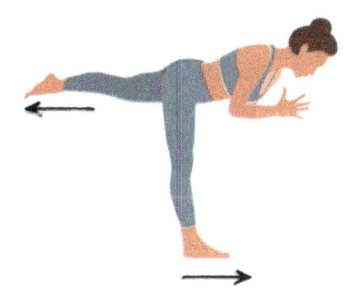

SEATED MEDITATION WITH DEEP BREATHING

⏱ 10 MINUTE MEDITATION

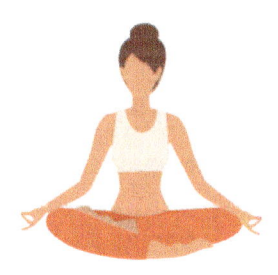

Chapter 7: Overcoming Challenges and Maintaining Progress

Chapter 7 is dedicated to navigating the path of personal growth with resilience and determination. Within this journey, encountering obstacles is inevitable. Still, these challenges can become stepping stones to greater success with the right strategies. We delve into potential setbacks you might face in your journey toward harmonizing physical and emotional well-being, offering practical solutions to stay on track.

7.1 Common Obstacles and Strategies for Overcoming Them

1. **Loss of Motivation**: Motivation can wane due to repetitive routines, lack of visible progress, or the human tendency toward fluctuating interest and energy.
   - **Strategy**: *Set small, achievable goals* to create a sense of accomplishment. Celebrate these milestones, however minor. Regularly vary your routine to keep it exciting and engaging.

2. **Time Management Issues**: Finding time for somatic practices, mindfulness, and preparing nutritious meals can be challenging in a busy life.
   - **Strategy**: *Prioritize* your activities by *scheduling* them as non-negotiable appointments in your calendar. Explore practices that can integrate into your daily routines, such as mindful breathing during commuting or somatic stretches during breaks.

3. **Physical Plateaus or Injuries**: Progress in physical practices can plateau, or injuries might occur, leading to frustration and setbacks.
   - **Strategy**: Listen to your body and adjust your practices accordingly. Incorporate rest and recovery, and consult

professionals as needed. Progress is not always linear; sometimes, rest is part of the journey.

4. Nutritional Challenges: Sticking to nutritional goals can take time, especially with conflicting information and the temptation of less healthy options.
- **Strategy**: Focus on whole, nutrient-dense foods that support your somatic practice. Plan meals to avoid impulsive eating, and allow yourself occasional treats to maintain balance and avoid feeling deprived.

5. Emotional and Mental Blocks: Doubts, fear of failure, or past traumas can impede your willingness to fully engage with somatic exercises or hinder your ability to maintain dietary changes.
- **Strategy**: Incorporate mindfulness and journaling to explore these emotional challenges. Consider seeking support from a therapist or counselor to work through deeper issues.

6. Social Pressure and Isolation: Feeling out of sync with friends or family due to lifestyle changes can lead to isolation.
- **Strategy**: Communicate openly about your goals and the importance of this journey. Seek communities or groups with similar interests to build a new support network.

Overcoming obstacles is not just about individual resilience but also about the strength found in the community. Whether it's family, friends, or like-minded individuals, having a support system can encourage and share in your successes and offer perspective when challenges arise. This chapter underscores that the journey towards harmonizing physical and emotional well-being, while personal, does not have to be solitary. Cultivating connections that nurture and support your goals can illuminate your path, making the journey more manageable and enriching.

A community of support on your journey to harmonized physical and emotional well-being plays a critical role. A strong support system can be the foundation of your success, offering encouragement, sharing insights, and providing much-needed motivation during difficult times.

7.2 Building a Support System
The Importance of a Support Network

Understanding the Value: At its core, a support system offers more than just company on your journey. It provides a sounding board for your experiences, advice when you face dilemmas, and a source of unconditional encouragement. Whether it's friends who share your passion for mindful living, family members who cheer on your efforts, or a community of practitioners who offer insights and advice, each uniquely bolsters your resolve and enriches your journey.

Creating Your Network: Building a support system might start with turning to those already in your life who understand and respect your commitment to bettering yourself through somatic practices and mindful nutrition. If your immediate circle is less familiar with your pursuits, look beyond:
- **Join Online Communities:** Digital platforms offer myriad groups dedicated to somatic practices, mindfulness, and nutrition. Here, you can share experiences and advice.
- **Attend Workshops and Classes**: Participating in workshops or classes deepens your practice and connects you with others who share your interests. These spaces can foster meaningful relationships built on shared experiences and mutual goals.
- **Seek Professional Support**: Professionals such as nutritionists, fitness trainers, or wellness coaches can offer tailored advice and become integral to your support network, guiding you with expertise and encouragement.

Leveraging Your Support System

Communicate Openly: Share your goals, challenges, and successes with your support network. Open communication can

give you different perspectives, valuable feedback, and increased accountability.
Offer Support in Return: Building a support system is a two-way street. Be there for your network members just as they are for you. Offering encouragement and being positive in others' journeys can reinforce your commitment to your goals.
Celebrate Together: Take the time to celebrate big and small milestones with your support system. These celebrations can reinforce the positive aspects of your journey and strengthen the bonds within your community.

Your support system becomes a cornerstone in maintaining the enthusiasm and commitment necessary for long-term success. The encouragement, accountability, and shared wisdom a support network provides can be instrumental in overcoming plateaus, revitalizing your motivation during periods of stagnation, and inspiring continued growth and learning. It reminds us that while the journey to wellness is personal, it need not be solitary. Through the collective strength of a support system, sustaining motivation and achieving lasting results becomes a possibility and a reality.

7.3 Sustaining Motivation and Results

We have almost reached the end of the book. We must mention the importance of delving into the essence of the longevity of your wellness journey, emphasizing strategies for maintaining weight loss and nurturing emotional well-being over time. This segment is critical to moving from a period of intense focus and change to integrating these practices into the fabric of your daily life.

Maintaining the progress you've achieved requires a blend of consistency, adaptability, and self-compassion. Here, we explore long-term strategies that empower you to sustain your motivation and the results you've worked hard to attain.
Establishing Sustainable Habits

Consistency Over Perfection: Embrace routines that fit seamlessly into your life, making consistency more achievable than perfection.

Regular somatic practice, even for just a few minutes a day, can have profound effects over time.

Mindful Eating as a Lifestyle: Rather than strict diets, focus on mindful eating—listening to your body's hunger cues, enjoying meals without distraction, and choosing foods that nourish both body and mind.

Adapting to Life's Changes

- **Flexible Mindset**: Acknowledge that life's circumstances change, and your wellness practices must adapt. Be open to modifying your routines while keeping your core goals in sight.
- **Continuous Learning**: Stay engaged by exploring new somatic exercises, mindfulness techniques, and nutritional insights. This not only prevents monotony but also deepens your understanding and commitment.

Fostering Emotional Resilience

- **Reflective Practices**: Regular journaling or meditative practices encouraging reflection can help maintain emotional balance. They offer a space to process experiences, celebrate achievements, and strategize around obstacles.
- **Seek Challenges**: Set new goals that challenge you physically and mentally. Whether mastering a more complex somatic sequence or trying a meditation retreat, new challenges keep the journey exciting and rewarding.

Building and Leaning on Your Community

- **Support Networks**: Continue to engage with your support system. Sharing your journey, exchanging ideas, and offering encouragement can reinforce your commitment and provide fresh perspectives.

- **Professional Guidance**: Periodic check-ins with wellness professionals can offer new insights, help reassess goals, and adjust strategies to align with your evolving needs.

Integrating Practices into Daily Life

As we approach the "Conclusion: Integrating Somatic Practices into Daily Life," the focus shifts to how the principles and practices explored throughout the book can become integral components of your daily routine. The goal is not just to sustain your progress but to elevate your overall quality of life.

- **Incorporate Movement into Daily Activities**: Find ways to integrate somatic movements into your everyday tasks. This could mean performing stretches while watching TV or practicing mindfulness during breaks at work.
- **Nutritional Mindfulness**: Make conscious food choices a natural part of meal planning and preparation, reflecting the nutritional principles that support your somatic practice and overall well-being.
- **Embrace Mindfulness in Everyday Moments**: Cultivate an attitude of mindfulness in all aspects of life, from how you engage with others to how you approach challenges.

In conclusion, sustaining motivation and results is more than just discipline; it's about lifelong commitment to your well-being. By integrating somatic practices, mindful living, and nutritional awareness into your daily life, you create a holistic approach to health that supports physical fitness and emotional balance and a deeply satisfying way of life.

Conclusion

Creating a Sustainable Routine

Creating a sustainable routine seamlessly integrating somatic exercises and mindful practices into everyday life is essential for long-term wellness. Creating a Sustainable Routine provides practical tips for making somatic exercises and mindfulness an integral part of your lifestyle, fostering a continuous connection to your physical and emotional well-being.

Start Small and Build Gradually

Begin by incorporating short, manageable practices into your daily routine. A five-minute morning meditation or a series of gentle pelvic clocks upon waking can set a positive tone for the day. As these practices become habitual, they gradually increase their duration and complexity.

Designate Specific Times for Practice

Consistency is key to forming lasting habits. Schedule specific times for your somatic exercises and mindfulness practices, just as you would for any important appointment. Early morning may work best for some, offering a quiet time for reflection and movement before the day's demands begin. For others, evening practices can serve as a soothing transition to rest.

Integrate Mindfulness into Routine Activities

Practice mindful eating by paying attention to your food's flavors, textures, and sensations. Turn mundane tasks, like washing dishes or walking, into opportunities for mindfulness by fully engaging with the experience and noticing every detail and feeling.

Use Reminders and Prompts

In our busy lives, forgetting our intentions to practice is easy. Leaving notes in visible places or setting reminders on your phone can prompt you to take mindful breaths, stretch, or check in with your body and emotions throughout the day.

Create a Dedicated Space

A specific area in your home for somatic practice can enhance your routine's sustainability. This doesn't need to be an ample space—just a quiet corner where you can roll out a yoga mat or meditate without interruptions. This physical space can serve as a visual cue, encouraging you to engage in your practice.

Adapt Practices to Fit Your Life

Your routine should complement your lifestyle, not complicate it. If you're short on time, consider integrating somatic movements during short breaks at work or practicing mindfulness while commuting. The key is to find opportunities within your existing schedule rather than seeing practice as an additional burden.

Connect with a Community

Joining a group—online or in-person—that shares your interest in somatic practices and mindfulness can provide motivation and inspiration. Sharing experiences and tips with others can introduce new perspectives and encourage consistency.

Reflect and Adjust Regularly

Periodically reflect on your routine and its impact on your well-being. What's working well? What could be improved? Flexibility is crucial; don't hesitate to adjust your practices to suit your evolving needs and circumstances better.

Celebrate Your Progress

Acknowledge the effort you've put into integrating somatic exercises and mindfulness into your daily life. Celebrating your progress, no matter how small, can reinforce the value of your practice and motivate you to continue.

By thoughtfully incorporating somatic exercises and mindful practices into your everyday life, you create a sustainable routine that supports your physical health and overall well-being. This holistic approach allows you to navigate life's challenges with greater ease, resilience, and presence, embodying the principles of somatic wellness in every action and moment.

The Journey Ahead

As we near the close of this enlightening journey through somatic practices, mindful living, and nutritional awareness, it's paramount to recognize that this experience marks not an end but the dawn of a profound, lifelong journey of self-discovery and well-being. "The Journey Ahead" is a testament to the enduring path you've embarked upon—a path paved with growth, learning, and an ever-deepening connection to oneself.

The Beginning, Not the End

You've navigated through the principles of somatic exercises, the tranquility of mindful practices, and the vitality of nutritional insights, fostering a more harmonious relationship between your body and mind. This journey, rich in discoveries and transformations, is the foundation of what will come. The practices you've learned and the changes you've initiated are the seeds of a flourishing garden of well-being that will grow and evolve with you over time.

Embracing Lifelong Learning

The essence of this journey lies in the understanding that self-discovery and well-being are not destinations but continuous processes. The landscape of our lives constantly changes, presenting new challenges, opportunities, and insights. Embracing a mindset of lifelong learning allows you to adapt and evolve your practices, ensuring they remain relevant and supportive as you navigate the varied terrains of life. Open-minded, curious, and willing to explore new dimensions of somatic practices and wellness philosophies.

Cultivating Resilience and Flexibility

As you move forward, you'll undoubtedly encounter obstacles and setbacks. However, the resilience you've built through somatic awareness and mindfulness equip you with the strength to face these challenges head-on. Obstacles are an opportunity for learning and growth. Flexibility in your approach—whether adjusting your routine, exploring new practices, or modifying your goals—will be your greatest ally in sustaining progress and well-being.

Nurturing Connections

The journey of well-being is enriched by the connections we foster—with ourselves and others. Continue to cultivate a supportive community that shares your values and aspirations. These connections provide encouragement, inspiration, and a sense of belonging, amplifying the joy and fulfillment derived from your practices.

The Role of Self-Compassion

At the heart of sustaining this journey is self-compassion. Be kind and patient with yourself, recognizing that growth often comes in waves, with its highs and lows. Celebrate your victories, learn from your experiences, and remember to treat yourself with the same level of compassion that you would offer to a dear friend. This self-compassion is the bedrock upon which enduring well-being is built.

Integrating Practices into Daily Life

As you continue on this path, seek ways to integrate somatic exercises, mindful practices, and nutritional insights into the fabric of your daily life. Let these practices naturally express your commitment to well-being, seamlessly woven into your routines, decisions, and interactions.

A Journey Without End

The journey ahead is infinite, filled with limitless potential for growth, discovery, and joy. Each day offers a new canvas to paint your experiences, guided by the practices and principles you've embraced. This book is but a map to start you on your way; the path you carve will be uniquely yours, a reflection of your courage, curiosity, and commitment to a life of harmonious well-being.

Remember, the journey of self-discovery and well-being is not a race but a lifelong stroll through the gardens of your existence. Each step reveals more about who you are, what you value, and how you wish to live. This is the beginning of a beautiful journey that promises not just a destination of well-being but a way of being in the world.

I hope this book has helped you on your path to wellness and offered insights into the wonderful synergy between movement, mindfulness and nutrition. If so, I invite you to share your experience. A **review on Amazon**, possibly positive, would be greatly appreciated. Your feedback supports the book and connects to a community of fellow travelers who share light and encouragement with one another.

I hope your journey is filled with discovery, health and happiness. May you find balance in movement, peace in stillness and nourishment in every choice.

The End ☺

Download your exercise and tracking journal if you haven't done so yet.

Last important thing before you say goodbye, don't forget to **leave** a, hopefully positive, **REVIEW** of the book. Reviews are crucial for us authors and for future readers.

You can download the journal via QR code:

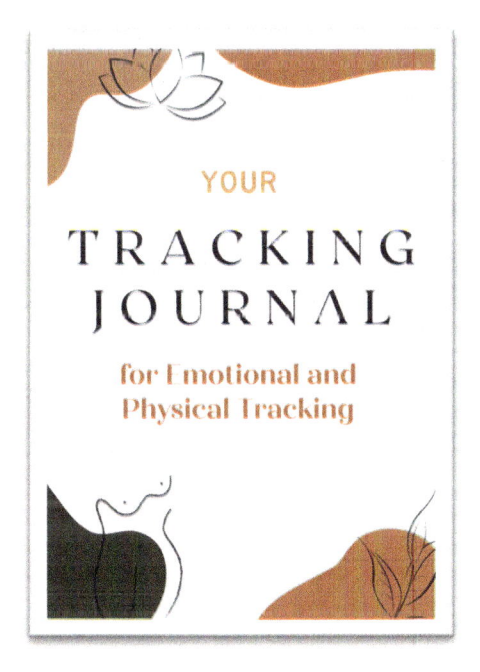

Printed in Great Britain
by Amazon